Nutritional Assessment

Suzanne Kitts

Nutritional Assessment

Solving the Individual Puzzle

Springer

Suzanne Kitts
Applied Exercise Science/Nutrition
Gannon University
Erie, PA, USA

Editorial Contact: Paige Ripperger

ISBN 978-3-032-22505-4 ISBN 978-3-032-22506-1 (eBook)
https://doi.org/10.1007/978-3-032-22506-1

This Springer imprint is published by the registered company Springer Nature Switzerland AG

The registered company address is: Gewerbestrasse 11, 6330 Cham, Switzerland

Preface

The development of *Nutritional Assessment: Solving the Individual Puzzle* began in 2003, as the author compiled information and crafted case studies to support both graduate and undergraduate students. Drawing from a range of textbooks and sources, the goal was to create a comprehensive resource that brings together all the essential components of nutritional assessment, something few texts offer in a single volume.

This textbook is designed to meet the educational needs of healthcare and wellness professionals, equipping them to guide patients, clients, and the public in understanding the connection between diet and health outcomes. It covers foundational knowledge and terminology, introduces key assessment concepts, explores practical applications, and includes case studies that encourage critical thinking and meaningful discussion.

As the healthcare field continues to evolve through ongoing research and discovery, this text aims to streamline complex information into an accessible format. There is an immense amount of information on how nutritional assessments could be done. Focusing on the essential pieces permits students and professionals to explore the intersections of the information. The textbook focuses on three core questions: *What* is the nutritional assessment process? *Who* comprises the healthcare team and benefits from assessment? and *How* can data collection be tailored to the individual?

Each chapter builds upon these guiding principles, helping students develop the skills to conduct assessments from the initial health history to completing recommendations derived from collected and analyzed data. Whether you're a student new to nutritional assessment or a seasoned practitioner seeking to broaden your expertise, this text offers a unique blend of classroom-ready instruction and professional development. Its step-by-step approach to energy equations allows for both comparison and flexibility, ensuring results can be adapted to individual needs. Through case studies and guided discussions, readers will strengthen their ability to think critically and connect assessment findings to overall health.

The author extends heartfelt gratitude to the faculty and peers whose support, guidance, and thoughtful feedback were instrumental in shaping this textbook. Special appreciation is given to Nutrition majors Lily Cunningham and Abigail Watts, whose insightful suggestions and keen observations helped identify areas for expansion and refinement, particularly within the case studies to better support student learning. Their contributions exemplify the essential role of student input in the development of educational resources, and the author remains deeply thankful for their involvement.

Erie, PA, USA Suzanne Kitts

Contents

Introduction to Nutritional Assessment 1

Abstract

The process of nutritional assessment is a unique process that can be complex due to the interaction between physiological, pathological, and psychosocial factors. It is important to gather a wide range of information like dietary and medical histories, anthropometric measures, and estimates of energy requirements, which will allow the team of health care professionals to best help individuals. This chapter will provide the basis of "why" the comprehensive data must be required. Additionally, a discussion about body composition or shape and health outcomes will be highlighted as these can be key indicators of an individual's health status. Nutritional needs will vary dramatically, and there is no single test that will fit all populations. The nutritional assessment is an ongoing process that the individual and health care professionals can continually assess for the best individual outcomes.

Keywords

Nutritional assessment · Dietary intake · Individualization · Somatotyping · Metabolic rate · Body composition · Health outcomes · Interdisciplinary collaboration

S. Kitts, *Nutritional Assessment*,
https://doi.org/10.1007/978-3-032-22506-1_1

Learning Objectives
By the end of this chapter, students should be able to:

- Explain the role of nutritional assessment in evaluating overall health and identifying risks for malnutrition and disease.
- Describe how nutritional assessment supports individuals' health guidance and behavior change.
- Identify and differentiate the four major components of a nutritional assessment:
  - medical history/dietary intake, anthropometrics, biochemical tests, and clinical signs/symptoms.
- Compare the scope of practice between clinical nutrition assessments and general health professional assessments.
- Analyze how body shape and genetic predispositions may influence health outcomes and nutritional needs.

Nutritional assessment is a key component to consider when connecting diet and nutrition to the overall health of an individual. However, where does one start? Then, once data is collected, how do we tailor the information for an individual so they can implement change? The purpose of this text is to show the processes of evaluating dietary intake, nutritional status of individuals, and relating health factors to possible disease states and outcomes. Ultimately, learning the difference between assessment methods, considering population standards, and individualizing assessments will be appropriate and purposeful for an individual.

Why Assess Nutrition?

Health care providers of all professional backgrounds can benefit from assessing nutritional status of individuals to discover four main areas: overall health, presence of malnutrition, predisposition to disease states or health-related factors (such as obesity, diabetes…), and how to provide guidance on achieving health goals. These are crucial areas as identifying risks for long-term health can be addressed to further the understanding of how diet and nutritional choices can make an impact. Education therefore becomes an essential piece of the individualized nutrition/health puzzle. Specifically, registered dietitians, nutritionists, physicians, physician assistants, and fitness professionals can provide an important link between diet, healthy eating habits, and lifestyle. Empowering individuals with knowledge that is found from assessments can connect the importance of balanced nutrition and lowering the risk of developing health issues. Let's examine the types of nutritional assessments professional providers will use in their realms.

Health Care Providers Uses of Dietary Assessments

Clinical Nutritional Assessment Health professionals such as registered dietitians (RDs) would be considered the specialists in this type of assessment. However, nurses, physicians, physician assistants, and occupational therapists can utilize nutritional assessments in the care of their patients. Health professionals can work in conjunction with RDs to fully assess and collaborate to monitor patients' nutritional status and identify risk factors.

Dietitians are educated and trained to utilize the Nutrition Care Process (NCP) to collect, investigate, and evaluate an individual's health care outcomes. The NCP provides a structured framework for dietitians to identify nutrition-related problems and their root causes. Depending on the population the dietician is working with, the NCP creates a model or workflow system that can be used individually or within a specific population. There are four distinct parts to the NCP model: nutrition assessment, nutrition diagnosis, nutrition intervention, and nutrition monitoring and evaluation. This multilayered model has a specific point of view that should be considered in the overall nutrition evaluation; a brief description of each can help see the benefit of this kind of model.

- At the core of this model is the individual or group/population that will be working with the nutrition professional. Everything surrounding the core will help the relationship of individual and nutrition professionals and establish the path forward through the assessment.
- The next layer surrounding the core has the four distinct parts that a nutrition professional will use to assess the individual's diet. The nutrition assessment, nutrition diagnosis, nutrition intervention, and nutrition monitoring and evaluation will be key in identifying, evaluating, planning, and assessing patient outcomes. These four specific areas of inquiry will help to individualize the needs or goals of the patient.
- The third ring of the NCP model shows the skills and abilities of RDs and nutrition professionals specifically from other health professionals. Clearly designating the expertise of dietetic knowledge that can be given to individuals that incorporates the most current knowledge and science regarding nutrition. Nutrition professionals adhere to their professional code and seamlessly collaborate with other health professionals to determine the best practices for the individual or population.
- The final outer ring of the NCP Model describes how the individual will receive nutrition information in various settings. Where the nutrition information comes from could vary from practice/health care systems to economic/social systems. Each of these settings can further individualize nutrition information as it would consider knowledge, values, educational level, and economic impact on nutrition.

RDs are an essential piece of overall nutritional assessment through their knowledge base and evidence-based advice and support. Working collaboratively with other health care professionals can ensure a comprehensive approach to nutrition. Therefore, the importance of a team approach can support a medical diagnosis, consider differential diagnoses, strategies for treatment, and recovery outcomes. There are four key components for clinical nutritional assessment:

1. Medical history and dietary intake evaluation—In this component, health professionals will review conditions like diabetes, heart disease, or gastrointestinal disorders that may affect nutrition and absorption of nutrients. In addition, information on eating habits, food preferences, allergies, and intolerances can be examined. A detailed history can provide a snapshot into an individual's current food and nutritional intake values, as well as behaviors related to diet.
2. Anthropometric measurements—Measuring height, weight, body mass index (BMI), and other physical measurements are used to assess and understand an individual's health status. Body size and distribution of mass can be measured via waist circumference and hip circumference, which can contribute to increased risk for cardiovascular disease factors related to abdominal obesity. Body composition will assess amounts of fat mass and fat-free mass throughout the body via skinfold measurements, bioelectrical impedance analysis, and advanced techniques such as hydrostatic weighing, dual-energy X-ray absorptiometry (DXA), and air displacement plethysmography (ADP). These techniques can detail excessive body fat in the midsection or viscera that could increase the risk of heart disease, diabetes, and certain cancers.
3. Biochemical tests—There are two subtypes of biochemical tests that can help to identify nutrient deficiencies, imbalances, and nutrient levels found in blood, urine, and stool samples. Static tests will measure the nutrient levels, various metabolites, and biomarkers in present or past intake. An example of static tests could include measuring serum iron levels or blood glucose levels to assess insulin resistance or diabetes. Functional tests will assess the function of the nutrient-dependent enzymes or physiological body processes of nutrient availability. For example, measuring hemoglobin to indicate iron status or changes in enzyme activity due to zinc deficiency.

4. Clinical symptoms and signs of malnutrition or deficiencies—This group of biochemical tests can help to identify nutrient deficiencies before the manifestation of clinical signs or symptoms develops. In some cases, deficiencies could develop slowly due to where they are stored in the bodily tissues. For example, vitamin A is a fat-soluble vitamin that is stored mostly in the liver; therefore, the physical development of a deficiency could take months to years. Therefore, a vitamin A deficiency can be indicated in skin health, where the manifestation could range from pale skin presentation to dry or flaky skin. Manifestation of deficiencies will happen once the body's stores have been depleted, and earlier diagnosis is beneficial.

Application for clinical nutritional assessment with health care professionals is important in managing chronic diseases to support recovery of post-surgical or illnesses. Using the four identified components will provide valuable information on an individual's current health status, developing treatment plans, and potentially improving the patient's outcomes.

Fitness and Sports Nutritional Assessment An assessment that contains the additional component of physical activity or exercise performance will need to consider the caloric impact of the activity. Professionals in fitness and sports nutrition can use nutritional assessments; however, they cannot prescribe any dietary specifics nor diagnose any nutritional diet issues. Therefore, the assessment will focus on enhancing performance by optimizing dietary choices through education to support the individual calorically. There are four components in this nonclinical nutritional assessment:

1. Energy balance analysis—A fitness professional will need to determine the individual's daily caloric needs versus actual intake. The caloric equilibrium, calories in versus calories out, can be a descriptive to visualize weight gain, weight loss, and no change in weight. The first step is to evaluate an individu-

al's metabolic rate and then determine the energy expenditure during physical activity. Once physical activity calories are determined, adjustments for the goal of weight gain, loss, or no weight gain can be implemented.

2. Macronutrient distribution—The macronutrients of carbohydrates, protein, and fat are needed to supply the body with sources of energy for physical activity. There are guidelines for health and fitness professionals to use for macronutrients that give a percentage of calories for an individual's diet. The framework for the macronutrient distribution is called Acceptable Macronutrient Distribution Range (AMDR), where 45–65% carbohydrates, 20–35% from fat, and 10–35% protein [1]. The AMDR has linked healthy dietary nutrient distribution to reducing the risk of chronic diseases like heart disease, diabetes, and certain cancers. The manipulation of these distribution ranges to support physical activity varying in state of training, intensity, and time. For example, carbohydrates are the main fuel for endurance and higher-intensity exercise. Protein is essential for repairing and growth of muscle tissue, and fats will provide long-term energy at lower intensity levels.
3. Hydration status—Monitoring hydration during physical activity is necessary and based on individual sweat loss and activity level. Evaluating electrolytes such as sodium and potassium can help prevent cramps and fatigue. Proper hydration is also essential for overall health, regulating body temperature, and transporting nutrients throughout the body. In addition, hydration can help differentiate an individual's thirst and hunger. Dehydration therefore can disrupt several systems and impede physical activity.
4. Assessment of micronutrient needs for performance and recovery—A full assessment of micronutrients and calories needed can improve performance and recovery. The assessment should include an examination of vitamins and minerals provided through a variety of sources in the natural diet. If there are missing micronutrients either due to lower calorie intake, overtraining, or low variety in diet, a personalized sup-

plementation plan can be formed. Education around micronutrient sources helps to make connections between diet, activity, and overall health.

Application of this type of assessment will focus on the relationship of calories, dietary variety, and physical activity. Tailoring nutritional plans for athletes and active individuals that will optimize muscle growth, endurance, and overall fitness is essential. Additionally, opportunities to educate individuals on preventing nutrient deficiencies and lack of variety or total calories will hinder performance.

Common Essential Nutritional Assessment for All Professionals The differences between clinical and general health professional nutritional assessments boil down to the scope of practice. The framework or boundaries for clinical assessment is established to systematically assess, identify, and diagnose malnutrition and disease states. Whereas general health professionals can use education, training, and advice on the role of food, calories, and dietary supplements that can help achieve proper nutrition. The difference between what the two professional types can do for assessment is clear; however, teaming together benefits the individual or patient. A combined approach promotes long-term health and well-being and a larger community of support for an individual. This common area also has key components that should be considered:

1. Dietary habits—Collecting information in either setting should include an in-depth examination of habits within a daily diet such as meal frequency, variety in diet, and portion sizes. Portion sizing and control is an under-utilized investigative tool to teach individuals appropriate serving sizes and the correlation to potential calories. Another area of investigation is determining snacking behaviors: processed versus whole foods, portions and timing of snacks, and mindful versus distracted eating. Assessing these behaviors can be helpful for the professional and the individual on eating habits and what might need to be adjusted.

2. Understanding nutritional needs based on age, lifestyle, and health conditions—The nutritional needs of an individual will vary based on the factors of age, sex, lifestyle, and corresponding health conditions. For example, protein requirements will increase in times of growth, increased physical activity, injury, and disease. All professions can then tailor dietary recommendations based on the individual's personal needs and health outcomes.
3. Identifying unhealthy dietary patterns—An assessment of the diet will also yield information on the number of added sugars, processed foods, and potential lack of nutrients. Items such as these can contribute to caloric increases and changes in nutrient availability. Additionally, large amounts of excessive sugar intake and processed foods could lead to various health issues, including obesity, diabetes, and heart disease. Once these unhealthy dietary patterns are identified, professionals can suggest healthier alternatives or substitutions that can align with their health outcomes.

The application of these components will be the connection between the clinical and general health professionals and will fully assess individual nutrition. The information gathered will help to educate individuals on maintaining a balanced diet, preventing lifestyle-related health conditions, and encouraging better dietary habits. This is a benefit of professionals sharing and collaborating on a comprehensive assessment to then provide tailored guidance for individuals that are seeking to achieve specific health goals.

Connecting Nutritional Assessment with Physical Findings

The use of dietary assessment can be useful to develop a picture of an individual's nutrient intake habits, dietary patterns, and potential for nutrient deficiencies or excesses. The assessment can be made more robust with the addition of physical findings and physiological states. An individual's body shape, fat distribution, and fat-free mass can play a critical role in health too.

Body Shape and Health Outcomes Body shape or types can be indicative of genetic makeup and potential predispositions to build muscle or store fat. First, understanding the classifications of somatotype theories will provide insight into an individual's build and composition. In the 1940s a body typing system was developed by W.H. Sheldon in which he connected body types to personality traits and criminal behavior. More recent research leans more into the body shapes' correlation to the overall relevance to health outcomes and metabolic risk [2]. There are three body types: endomorphy, mesomorphy, and ectomorphy [3].

1. Endomorphy—This body type is characterized by a great presence of fatty tissue, curvy or rounded shape, larger frame, and lower muscle content. Some research has suggested that individuals who are endomorphs have a slower metabolism, which could lead to easier weight gain and make it harder to lose weight once it is stored. Individuals that display this classification may also be at an increased risk for metabolic syndrome, type 2 diabetes, and cardiovascular disease.
2. Mesomorphy—In contrast, this body type is characterized by having an athletic build, efficient metabolism, and greater muscularity over fatty tissue. With the presence of more muscle, individuals are more active, which may reduce their risk of some metabolic disorders.
3. Ectomorphy—These individuals are characterized by a lean and thin build with low body fat and low muscle mass. Research has stated that these individuals may have faster metabolisms and have trouble with gaining and maintaining weight. Nutritional interventions such as high-calorie diets and increases in physical activity might not encourage weight gain too. Individuals that display this classification may be susceptible to nutritional deficiencies.

Ultimately, understanding these somatotypes is a factor influencing an individual's health or potential predispositions. However, this classification should be used as a guideline and not a defining factor of health status. Other factors such as lifestyle choices, genetics, and environmental considerations should be factored in combination with a nutritional assessment.

Secondly, research has shown that obesity related to morbidity and mortality can be associated with higher fat accumulation in bodily tissue [4]. The body shapes are determined by the distribution of weight and fatty tissues around the abdomen. The health implication of visceral or central fat around the abdomen is associated with increased risk of heart disease, diabetes, and metabolic syndrome. There are two associated body shapes that could have potential negative health outcomes:

1. Android or apple-shaped: Individuals that display this type of body shape will accumulate fat tissue around the midsection or central trunk region, referred to as visceral adipose tissue (VAT). The distribution of fat can be found in the chest, abdomen, and arms, thereby increasing the risk factors for various health risks of heart disease and diabetes. The mechanism of the fat in and around the central trunk causes fat to build around the liver, heart, and arteries, releasing free fatty acids and inflammatory markers into the bloodstream. This inflammation process disrupts the normal metabolic process, which can lead to insulin resistance. This disruption of the metabolic process causes further damage to the arteries and organs. Additionally, genetics and individual lifestyle factors, such as diet and physical activity, should be considered in determining the overall risk for metabolic syndrome outcomes (Fig. 1.1).
2. Gynoid or pear-shaped: This fat distribution can be characterized by accumulation of fatty tissue in the periphery of the body. The increase of subcutaneous fat in the hips, buttocks, and thighs, or peripheral obesity, does not have an increased risk of cardiovascular disease like android fat. Gynoid fat can still contribute to overall health issues such as orthopedic problems in the hip, knee, and other joints due to increased weight. However, the mechanism of the fat distribution to the periphery has a decreased correlation link to cardiovascular disease when compared to android fat distribution.

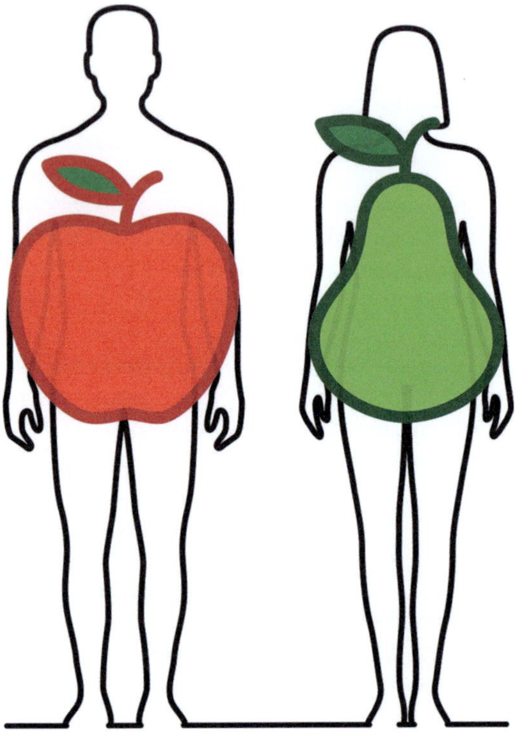

Fig. 1.1 Fat distribution—central or android (apple) versus periphery or gynoid (pear)

Expanding the assessment to include physical stature or somatotyping can be beneficial when determining possible health outcomes for an individual. By recognizing how fat distribution can influence metabolism and nutritional needs, health professionals can refine dietary recommendations. More specifically, the value of including physical stature and somatotyping can be incorporated in several ways:

Tailored Energy Requirements The theory of somatotyping can hold a piece of the puzzle when it comes to the influence of metabolic rate. It is proposed that ectomorphs, with leaner build, might require a higher caloric intake as noted by their faster metabolic nature. In contrast, mesomorphs, with muscular build, require a balanced caloric intake of all micronutrients to supply energy and support active energy requirements. Professionals can ultimately optimize the macronutrient distributions and create nutritional strategies.

Enhanced Disease Risk Assessment Body composition and fat distribution correlate to increased negative health risks, especially in the visceral region. By considering how fat can be distributed, rather than just an individual's weight, the approach for health professionals will be tailoring dietary changes to support more effective weight management. The combination of nutritional assessment and body shape enhances the assessment while improving overall health outcomes.

Chapter Summary

Nutritional assessment can be a key method to assess an individual's health and risk factors for developing disease factors. Health care professionals together will evaluate dietary nutrients, biochemical markers, anthropometric measures, and the clinical signs of nutritional deficiencies. These approaches develop the groundwork for identifying and addressing nutritional imbalances that might impact overall health. Integrating the physical stature and body type of an individual will enhance the accuracy of the assessments as more data can provide a better understanding of the metabolic health and disease correlation. Ultimately, these steps are necessary for health care professionals to recommend an individual's physiological and metabolic health profile.

Chapter Review Questions

1. What is the primary purpose of conducting a nutritional assessment?
2. Compare the roles of clinical health professionals and general health professionals in conducting nutritional assessments. How do their scopes of practice differ?

3. What types of information are gathered during medical history and dietary intake evaluation?
4. Define anthropometric measurements and give three examples.
5. How can nutritional assessments empower individuals to make meaningful lifestyle changes?
6. In what ways might cultural, socioeconomic, or environmental factors influence the outcomes of a nutritional assessment?

References

1. IOM. Dietary reference intakes for energy, carbohydrate, fiber, fat, fatty acids, cholesterol, protein, and amino acids. Washington, DC: The National Academies Press; 2002/2005.
2. Galić BS, Pavlica T, Udicki M, Stokić E, Mikalački M, Korovljev D, Čokorilo N, Drvendžija Z, Adamović D. Somatotype characteristics of normal-weight and obese women among different metabolic subtypes. Arch Endocrinol Metab. 2016;60(1):60–5. https://doi.org/10.1590/2359-3997000000159. PMID: 26909484; PMCID: PMC10118907.
3. Bernard TJ. William Sheldon. Encyclopedia Britannica; 2024. https://www.britannica.com/biography/William-Sheldon
4. Fu J, Hofker M, Wijmenga C. Apple or pear: size and shape matter. Cell Metab. 2015;21(4):507–8, ISSN 1550-4131. https://doi.org/10.1016/j.cmet.2015.03.016.

2 Nutritional Assessment Terminology

Abstract

Learning key nutritional assessment terminology is critical for ensuring individuals' health outcomes are being met and enabling clear communication between the health care team. This chapter will explore and define several terms that will be utilized in this text as well as in the professional realm and research. Several of the definitions will use current key global agencies' categories as they share common frameworks for describing malnutrition, anthropometric indicators, and specific population-level indicators. Successful navigation and understanding of this terminology will equip readers with the language and tools necessary to interpret data accurately, apply evidence-based practices, and contribute effectively to both patient care and broader public health initiatives.

Keywords

Terminology · Anthropometry · Body composition · Population indicators · Evidence-based practice · Health outcomes

S. Kitts, *Nutritional Assessment*,
https://doi.org/10.1007/978-3-032-22506-1_2

Learning Objectives
By the end of this chapter, students should be able to:

- Explain the purpose and importance of understanding nutritional assessment terminology in professional and research settings.
- Describe how dietary recall methods, PAL, TDEE, and RDA contribute to evaluating an individual's nutritional needs.
- Interpret how metabolism, metabolic syndrome, and nutritional status relate to health outcomes.
- Analyze how terminology supports the interpretation of nutritional data for individualized diet planning.
- Identify conditions such as failure to thrive (FTT) and metabolic syndrome using appropriate terminology.

Developing an understanding of nutritional assessment requires knowledge of key terms and concepts that are used in research and professional settings. This chapter introduces essential terminology used in various areas to determine fundamental concepts to descriptions within populations. Increasing awareness and usage of these terms, health care professionals can better interpret nutritional data and then make decisions for individual diet planning. The terminology presented in this chapter will serve as a foundation for navigating nutritional assessment theories, methodologies, and interventions to achieve practical applications.

Anthropometry

Anthropometry refers to measuring and analyzing a person's physical dimensions. Derived from the Greek words "anthropos," meaning human, and "metron," meaning measure, anthropometry is commonly thought of as the study of human body measurements. The measurements that are utilized will assess the size, portions, and composition of the human body. This broad area of study can then benefit various professional fields that are not limited to health care; in fact, human measurements in ergonomic design, forensic science, and military and law enforcement can benefit from the data.

Specifically, in nutritional assessment, measurements that include weight, height, body circumferences, and more are beneficial to assess nutritional status and health. These measures help determine body composition and can provide insights into an individual's diet and nutritional intake. Anthropometric data can be used for several things, including evaluating growth patterns in children, assessing whether someone is underweight, overweight, or obese, monitoring changes in body composition over time, and estimating energy needs based on body size and composition. Tools such as scales, skinfold calipers, measuring tapes, and more can be combined with nutritional recall questionnaires to provide insight into an individual's nutritional health.

Basal Metabolic Rate (BMR)

Basal metabolic rate (BMR) is the number of calories needed to maintain basic physiological functions in the body at rest. This contains factors from breathing, circulation, and cell production. Ultimately, determining an individual's BMR will show the minimum energy needed to feed the body and maintain current weight at the basic level. Influences from factors such as age, height, weight, gender, genetics, and body composition will be considered in the total daily expenditure.

BMR relates to weight through the calories that are burned throughout the day. Essentially, if one intakes more calories (food) than they are putting out (activity), most likely an individual will gain weight. If one consumes less calories (food) and spends more calories (activity), an individual will lose weight. A balance of input and output of calories is ideal for maintaining a current weight. Therefore, BMR can be considered a baseline calculation of calories at rest, and then additional calories will be added for other metabolic processes and activity calories. Knowing an individual's BMR will be one piece of energy or calorie usage that will be important when it comes to weight management.

Finally, BMR is very individualized, and there is not a constant or "normal" standard that all individuals will be measured against. There are estimates for males and females; however, the other factors that were described above (age, height, weight…) become unique considerations for individuals to understand their caloric rate.

Bioavailability

Bioavailability focuses on the degree to which a nutrient from a food or supplement source will be absorbed and utilized in the body. For the nutrient to be utilized effectively, the rate and extent of absorption from the digestive system and then distribution for its intended purpose are key. This process is contingent on the nutrient proportion provided by the overall diet (sourced from diet or dietary supplement) that can be absorbed and then available for various physiological functions. If there are issues during this process, it may lead to malabsorption or deficiency of key nutrients.

There are several factors that affect a nutrient's bioavailability, including the chemical form, presence of other food components, age or health status of an individual, and presence of nutritional deficiencies. Here are some examples that can show the complexities of bioavailability:

- as we age, gastric acid declines thereby decreasing the ability to absorb micronutrients (individual factor)
- consuming vitamin C with nonheme iron can help improve its absorption (dietary interaction)
- protein availability will depend on the proportion of amino acids that are ingested to be utilized for protein synthesis and other metabolic fates
- the method of cooking (boiling versus steaming) or processing (physical breakdown or milling) can alter the availability of some micronutrients
- food–drug interactions can interfere with absorption by changing the gut flora, thereby decreasing the amount available to use or changing how they are processed

Body Mass Index (BMI)

Body mass index (BMI), developed by mathematician Lambert Adolphe Jacques Quetlet, is an equation that compares an individual's weight to their height. This provides a quick and inexpensive way to screen for obesity, or if an individual is over/underweight. BMI is used as apopulation health measure to study populations, which makes it not the most efficient measure to use for pregnant women or athletes because other factors such as muscle mass are not considered in this equation. It is important to understand that BMI only assesses the correlation between height/weight and the relationship between various chronic disease risks. BMI does not have the capacity to assess body fat percentage, muscle mass distribution, or the ability to distinguish between fat and muscle tissue.

BMI is calculated by dividing a person's weight in kilograms (kg) by their height in meters squared. The four common categories for BMI range from very underweight (under 18.5), healthy weight (18.5–24.9), overweight (25.0–29.9), and obese (over 30). However, in health care domestically and internationally, there are established categories or classifications which can make it confusing on which to use.

The Centers for Disease Control and Prevention (CDC) in the United States uses BMI as an easy method or tool to assess weight that is relative to height in a general population to monitor health [1]. There are two divisions: adults that are 20 years old and older and children to teens (2–19 years old). The adult standard weight status categories are used for men and women, and the categories can be seen below:

BMI	Weight status
Below 18.5	Underweight
18.5–24.9	Normal
25.0–29.9	Overweight
30.0 and above	Obese

BMI in children and adolescents will be interpreted differently; here BMI will be correlated to the subject's age and sex. This method is essential with this population due to growth patterns and changes in fat tissue that are experienced during childhood. Changing the way BMI is interpreted in children and adolescents will also introduce a classification based on percentiles specific to age that can be mapped through the growth cycle. The BMI-for-age percentile categories can be seen below:

Percentile ranking	Weight status
Less than 5th percentile	Underweight
5th percentile to less than 85th percentile	Healthy weight
85th percentile to less than 95th percentile	Overweight
Equal to or greater than the 95th percentile	Obese

The World Health Organization (WHO) also uses BMI to classify individuals for overweight and obesity risk. The WHO correlates being overweight with increased fat tissue deposits and additional health risks associated with obesity. The same calculation of weight (kg)/height^2 (m^2) is used with additional measurements or assessments that further justify an obesity diagnosis such as waist circumference or hip-to-waist ratio. The following breakdown for BMI categories will be designated by age and then a further breakdown by gender in infants, children, and adolescents [2].

Adults A BMI greater than or equal to 25 is overweight, and BMI greater or equal to 30 is obese. Additionally, the WHO classifies adult obesity into an additional category to account for population variations that may exist in other countries. Initially, the WHO was using data from predominantly White populations. Therefore, the inclusion of other ethnic groups will help to understand body fat distribution and higher health risks at potentially lower BMIs. The BMI WHO classifications or threshold for international use can be seen below:

BMI	Weight status
<18.5 kg/m^2	Underweight
18.5–24.9 kg/m^2	Normal weight
25.0–29.9 kg/m^2	Overweight
30.0–34.9 kg/m^2	Obesity (class I)
35.0–39.9 kg/m^2	Obesity (class II)
≥40 kg/m^2	Obesity (class III)

Children Under 5 Years of Age (utilizing the established WHO Child Growth Standards median charts and Tables)

- overweight is weight-for-height greater than 2 standard deviations above the standard median
- obesity is weight-for-height greater than 3 standard deviations above the standard median

Children Aged 5–19 Years (utilizing the established WHO Child Growth Standards median charts and Tables)

- overweight is BMI-for-age greater than 1 standard deviation above the standard median
- obesity is greater than 2 standard deviations above the standard median

Ultimately, BMI should be used as a population guideline for health status and as part of initial screening in health care assessments and evaluations. The CDC and WHO utilize BMI measurements as a reasonable indicator to evaluate overall body fat for overweight or obesity indicators for adults and children. As explained, BMI should not be solely used as a diagnostic tool and should implement other measurements that can assess body fat distribution. Other diagnostic tools will be discussed, and the importance of their use will help enhance the correlation of BMI, overall body fat distribution, and connection to chronic diseases.

Exercise Activity Thermogenesis (EAT) and Non-exercise Activity Thermogenesis (NEAT)

The calories that are utilized and burned through activity will be accounted to determine an individual's total daily calorie needs. Interestingly, there are two types of activity calories: the energy that is burned when an individual trains or works out, and the other focuses on the energy that is created in all other activities not related to training, eating, or sleeping.

EAT—energy calories that are in this category are specifically focused on activities that increase heart rate and breathing over time. Specifically, activities that are planned or structured such as running, weightlifting, cycling, and swimming. Regular physical activity may increase the body's ability to burn calories for this kind of activity.

NEAT—energy calories here are considered more general movements found throughout the day. Activities could include standing, brushing teeth, house chores, and even fidgeting or unconscious movements. This type of activity is important in total calories expended and therefore should be increased in individuals that have a sedentary lifestyle. For example, if an individual has a desk job, getting up every 50 minutes to walk around the office or taking stairs instead of an elevator will burn extra calories passively.

Dietary Recall Method

Dietary recall methods are techniques for health care professionals to collect information from individuals about their diet. These methods ask individuals to recount foods/beverages, portion sizes, cooking methods, and sometimes who they ate with or where they ate. Collection methods include food diaries, 24-h recall, three-to-five-day food journals, food frequencies, questionnaires, and computer-based or app programs. Data collected through these methods can help to assess dietary patterns, help to identify common food groups, and estimate nutrient intakes for the individual.

There are some considerations or issues that should be considered with recall methods. Self-reported diet recalls are widely used as they can show an individual's nutritional choices day-to-day, which can be very helpful. However, research has shown there can be inherent issues with the self-reporting of diets such as changing normal eating behaviors, underreporting or omission of nutrients, and minimizing overall caloric density [3]. More specifically, reliance on memory for the 24-h recall places the burden on the individual to remember all food consumed, and this is where the overestimate/underestimate of the portions can happen. Using a collection tool such as the food frequency questionnaires (FFQ) can be very useful for research data collection; however, it is labor intensive as it uses a Likert scale with up to 90+ questions. Tools like this introduce issues with interviewer/participant bias or educational/cultural factors such as lack of understanding or knowledge base, food insecurity, or literacy levels.

To decrease or mitigate concerns with self-reporting dietary information, there are several options to use as part of a nutritional assessment. First, having a trained interviewer that could lead an individual through their recall will help to improve the accuracy of diet information. Developing set methods that will employ memory aids through probing questions will help participants with follow-up sessions as they will understand what will need to be recalled. Next, the use of technology through computer programs and apps has provided easier access for individuals to record their diet. The dietary apps have grown from simple input of a meal to the ability of scanning UPC or barcodes of foods for direct input based off the information for that food item. Additionally, the apps can calculate total calories, macronutrient ratios, and recommended allowances for the individual, which is very important for overall learning and education about their diet. Finally, using a secondary collection instrument can help individuals recall and increase consistency of diet reporting.

Failure to Thrive

Failure to thrive (FTT) is when there is an unusual pattern in weight gain from the lack of insufficient available nutrition and is documented from the abnormal weight gain over time. This is also used to describe the patient who fails to meet the normal standards of growth based on adjusted gestational age and sex or if their weight drops at least two percentiles below the anticipated range on a standardized growth chart. There are four aspects that should be considered as part of FTT: inadequate total calorie intake, difficulty utilizing calories, weight faltering, and impact on growth. In essence, these aspects focus on the calories (consumption vs. ability to use) and the ability to grow or gain weight appropriately. Collecting information from these areas helps to build a holistic understanding of the possible problem signals in nutritional status.

Macronutrients

Macronutrients are the essential building blocks we need in larger quantities and provide the body with energy through calories and nutrients to maintain health. The three macronutrients are carbohydrates, fats, and protein, which are consumed through a balanced diet of all the nutrients. For the body to function daily, the macronutrients will need to support an individual's energy needs based on their weight, age, gender, and health status. The energy provided (calories) from each nutrient is as follows: Carbohydrate 4 g/cal, Fat 9 g/cal, and Protein 4 g/cal. Knowing the energy or calorie yield will help to estimate the total calories the individual will need. Additionally, there are established guidelines that individuals can follow to guide their consumption and maintain overall health. The Acceptable Macronutrient Distribution Range (AMDR) [4] suggests the following percentages:

- 45–65% Carbohydrates
- 20–35% Fats
- 10–35% Proteins

Micronutrients

Micronutrients are vitamins and minerals that are needed in smaller amounts (micrograms and milligrams) for vital functions in the body to maintain body functions, growth, and development. There is no energy associated with micronutrients; rather they will serve as coenzymes in energy production. There are also numerous factors that will influence the amounts of each micronutrient individual will need to maintain a healthy diet. The factors vary from person to person depending on the following factors (examples are included when needed):

- Physiological factors
  - Age and sex
  - Life stage (newborn, toddler, teenager, adult, elderly)
  - Physical activity (daily/weekly activity minutes or activities)
- Dietary factors
  - Food and diet patterns (fresh vs. processed, food choices, portion sizes, frequency, and timing)
  - Food preparation and/or processing (baking/frying/steaming)
  - Food availability and/or access (ability to obtain sufficient food or acquire nutritious food)
- Individual health factors
  - Underlying and chronic diseases (disease states can interfere with absorption and use of nutrients)
  - Genetic predispositions (cancers, diabetes, obesity, celiac diseases can affect nutrients)
  - Drug-nutrient interactions (some examples: antibiotics interfere with iron absorption, diuretics cause the increase of potassium)
- Other factors
  - Smoking (negatively impacts the ability to absorb essential vitamins and minerals)
  - Alcohol consumptions (inhibits the absorption of nutrients and provides empty calories that provide no positive calorie worth)

- Stress (can impact eating habits and dietary choices)
- Environmental impacts (decrease of farms, weather impacts, contamination of food sources)

Considering the above contributing factors will help individuals and health care providers assess micronutrient status and health needs [5].

Malnutrition

Malnutrition refers to a state where an individual's intake of nutrients is either deficient, excessive, or imbalanced. This leads to altered body composition and impacted physical function. This can manifest undernutrition, which refers to not having enough nutrients or overnutrition, which refers to too many nutrients. Malnutrition is analyzed by several factors such as weight, height, body composition, and dietary intake.

Malnutrition affects every organ system's function and recovery, such as muscle function, cardi-respiratory function, gastrointestinal function, immunity, and wound healing. Malnutrition can also result in psychological effects such as depression, anxiety, and self-neglect.

Clinically, malnutrition can be identified by a collection of symptoms ranging from unintentional weight loss, lack of appetite, fatigue, and loss of muscle strength. The World Health Organization adds the low weight-for-height designation to the definition to further diagnose children with malnutrition in designated populations.

Metabolism

The function of how your body turns to energy through the foods and drinks you consume that keep us alive and functioning. This is a chemical process that is continuously happening in the body through your cells. This function helps us breathe, enables us to have movement, heal and much more at rest and during activity.

Metabolism is not just about the calories we intake, which is metabolic rates which we will see in basal metabolic rate (BMR), but it is much more complex and this system functions with our body and plays a huge role in our health.

There are several factors that can influence metabolism that are important to consider managing weight and overall health. Here are some of the factors:

- Anthropometric measures: age, gender, body size, and body composition
- Activity level: physical activity will increase energy expenditure
- BMR: the amount of energy the body uses at rest for breathing/temperature/circulation

Metabolic Syndrome

Metabolic Syndrome refers to a group of health conditions including high blood pressure, high blood sugar, excess abdominal fat, and abnormal cholesterol levels. When presented together, it significantly increases the risk of cardiovascular disease and type 2 diabetes.

The diagnostic criteria look for at least three of five of the following factors:

- Increased waist circumference, which is measured at the level of the belly button, with specific cut-off points based on gender and ethnicity.
- High blood pressure with systolic blood pressure above 130 mmHg or diastolic blood pressure above 85 mmHg.
- High fasting blood sugar with a fasting glucose level above 100 mg/dL. High triglycerides with a triglyceride level above 150 mg/dL.
- Low HDL cholesterol below 40 mg/dL for men and below 50 mg/dL for women.

These potential risk factors individually can be managed with lifestyle modification through activity and dietary changes. However, when these conditions become additive or combine to three or more, a diagnosis of metabolic syndrome can be made. Reducing the risks by managing weight, increasing cumulative physical activity, and following focused diet that supports overall health will be positive for an individual.

Nutritional Status

Nutritional status consists of the evaluation of an individual's health by looking at diet, body mass, and biochemical data. Also using clinical indicators such as body mass, BMI, and unintentional weight loss. Assessing an individual's nutritional status can help to identify quality of life, potential disease prevention, and possible treatment outcomes.

Obesity

A chronic condition that is characterized as an individual that has an excessive accumulation of body fat tissue that has the potential to negatively impact their overall health. The excessive accumulation of fat tissue may impact several of the bodily systems, which can include the cardiovascular, respiratory, digestive, endocrine, skeletal, muscular, and nervous. The impact and disruption of these systems due to excessive fat tissue can be complex and detrimental to an individual. As weight increases, underlying health issues such as metabolic syndrome and mental health issues can increase.

Obesity is primarily identified using the Body Mass Index (BMI) and using waist circumference numbers. A BMI of 30 or higher is considered obese; see the above BMI definition. Waist circumference measurements are a way to assess regional fat distribution, and higher measurements indicate a greater risk for obesity related health issues. The National Center for Chronic Disease Prevention and Health Promotion uses the waist circumference values of 40 inches (102 cm) or more for men and 35 inches (88 cm) or more for women as "at risk" for obesity-related health issues. Managing/losing weight and working with a health care provider can help to reduce weight by just 5–10%, which can lower risk factors and improve overall health [6, 7].

Physical Activity Level (PAL)

Physical Activity Level (PAL) is used to show the daily activity calories as an estimate of a person's total expenditure (TEE). PAL quantifies the energy yielded from all activities, from everyday movements (household chores, going up stairs, and even fidgeting) to daily exercise. PAL does not include resting energy requirements (RER) or expenditure (REE), as this energy is reserved to maintain daily functions such as heart rate, breathing, and blood circulation. Although the resting energy is not included in PAL, it is needed as part of the ratio to find PAL.

$$\text{PAL} = \frac{\text{TEE}}{\text{REE}}$$

To determine PAL, it is helpful to categorize activity levels for common physical activities based on the activity's intensity, type, and duration of the activity. The levels of activity are sedentary, lightly active, moderately active, and very active. Within each of these activity levels, examples can be given to help understand specific activities that may be related to the level.

Sedentary	PAL 1.4–1.69	Desk job, minimal movement, light household chores
Light active	PAL 1.7–1.99	Walking at leisurely pace, light yard work
Moderate active	PAL 2.0–2.4	Brisk walking, playing paddleball
Very active	PAL 2.4+	Jogging, running, fitness classes that increase heart rate and breathing

This information can be used to assess overall health and then modify activities to meet fitness and health goals. Individuals that are identified as sedentary may be at risk for chronic diseases such as obesity, Type 2 diabetes, and cardiovascular disease.

Recommended Dietary Allowance (RDA)

The average daily intake of specific nutrients is considered sufficient to meet the needs of most healthy individuals based on age and gender of a population. This information can be used as a point of reference to see if an individual is getting enough of certain nutrients through their diet. Applying the RDA to analyze an individual's dietary intake can help to discover potential nutrient deficiencies or excesses and potentially design a personalized nutrition education. The RDA can be an adequate goal to maintain; some individuals may require certain nutrients depending on their circumstances such as age, gender, activity levels, and health/disease state.

Total Daily Energy Estimate (TDEE)

The calculation of TDEE is used to make an estimate of how much energy the body burns over a 24-h period and how many calories are needed. This is accomplished by using the findings in basal metabolic rate (BMR), activity levels (exercise activity thermogenesis (EAT) and non-exercise activity thermogenesis (NEAT)), and the thermic effect of food (TEF). The three contributors (BMR, EAT/NEAT, and TEF) can account for the total TDEE. The percentage breakdown of the three contributors is as follows: BMR 60–70%, EAT 5–10%, NEAT 15–20%, and TEF 7–10%. Please note that these percentages vary due to individual differences and research sources.

Determining one's TDEE can be beneficial in understanding how many calories they would need to either maintain, lose, and/or gain weight. There are several factors that can affect TDEE:

- Age and gender
- Activity level
- Body composition (size and weight)
- Disease state or illnesses
- Hormone levels
- Genetics

Chapter Summary

Having a foundational understanding of nutritional assessment terminology will be essential in effective communication, accurate diagnosis, and meaningful intervention in the field of nutrition and health. These terms serve as the shared language among professionals, enabling consistency in evaluating nutritional status, identifying risk factors, and developing personalized nutrition education. As you progress through each chapter, you will encounter these foundational terms and directly apply knowledge to dietary evaluations and clinical case studies. Let this terminology be your toolkit—empowering you to assess, advocate, and innovate with clarity and confidence.

Chapter Review Questions

1. What is the purpose of learning nutritional assessment terminology in health care and research settings?
2. Define anthropometry and explain its relevance in nutritional assessment.
3. Define metabolic syndrome and list the conditions associated with it.
4. What does Recommended Dietary Allowance (RDA) represent?
5. How might a health care professional use dietary recall methods to evaluate a client's nutritional status?
6. Provide an example of how understanding bioavailability might influence dietary recommendations.
7. In what ways does mastering nutritional terminology improve communication between health care professionals?

References

1. Centers for Disease Control and Prevention (U.S). Body mass index: considerations for practitioners. 2011. https://stacks.cdc.gov/view/cdc/25368.
2. Weir CB, Jan A. BMI classification percentile and cut off points. [Updated 2023 Jun 26]. In: StatPearls [Internet]. Treasure Island: StatPearls Publishing; 2025. Available from: https://www.ncbi.nlm.nih.gov/books/NBK541070/.
3. Subar AF, Freedman LS, Tooze JA, et al. Addressing current criticism regarding the value of self-reported dietary data. J Nutr. 2015;145(12):2639–45. https://doi.org/10.3945/jn.115.219634.
4. https://www.dietaryguidelines.gov/resources/2020-2025-dietary-guidelines-online-materials
5. https://www.ncbi.nlm.nih.gov/books/NBK597352/
6. Ryan DH, Yockey SR. Weight loss and improvement in comorbidity: differences at 5%, 10%, 15%, and over. Curr Obes Rep. 2017;6(2):187–94. https://doi.org/10.1007/s13679-017-0262-y. PMID: 28455679; PMCID: PMC5497590.
7. Kim D, Hou W, Wang F, Arcan C. Factors affecting obesity and waist circumference among US adults. Prev Chronic Dis. 2019;16:180220. https://doi.org/10.5888/pcd16.180220.

Anthropometric Measures and Application in Nutritional Assessment

3

Abstract

This chapter investigates estimated energy equations essential to individuals' factors that need to be considered before use. Due to the large number of possible equations, practitioners will need to determine which equation might be most appropriate. Additionally, for certain populations, estimation equations may under- or overestimate energy/calories needed due to the limited accuracy for individuals who are not within the "average" healthy population. Therefore, assessing patient-specific factors and understanding the equations strength to account for body composition, ethnicity, and possible disease states will increase the effectiveness of the equation. The more individual data points and combining the strength of an equation will allow for a more informed decision-making process for the nutritional assessment.

Keywords

Estimated energy equations · Patient-specific factors Anthropometric measures · Body composition · Metabolic rate Predictive accuracy · Nutritional status · Clinical interventions

S. Kitts, *Nutritional Assessment*,
https://doi.org/10.1007/978-3-032-22506-1_3

Learning Objectives

By the end of this chapter students should be able to:

- Identify key patient-specific factors (including age, body composition, ethnicity, gender, activity level, and disease state) that influence the accuracy and applicability of nutritional assessment formulas.
- Explain the limitations of common nutritional assessment equations and why they may under- or over-estimate energy needs in different populations.
- Analyze how anthropometric indices and stacked assessment methods improve predictive power and interpretation of nutritional data.
- Assess how combining multiple data sources enhances decision-making in nutritional assessment and supports individualized recommendations.

As previously defined, anthropometric measures will need to gather individual data points that will include height, weight, and possibly body circumferences. This information will provide quantifiable data that will be used to assess body size, composition, and growth patterns and ultimately reflect the individual's nutritional status. For example, an individual that presents with a high body mass index (BMI), measures overweight, and lives a sedentary lifestyle could indicate malnutrition and have an increased risk for metabolic syndrome. The next step would be to evaluate the data points or metrics for this individual to guide the clinical and dietary interventions. The application of the data collected by the measures will set the foundation for nutritional assessment. Therefore, it is important to understand how the anthropometric measures or applications will be utilized and valid for their use.

Considerations for Using Nutritional Assessment Equations

Patient-Specific Factors The first consideration in using the assessment equations, and an essential piece, is the patient-specific factors that can influence accuracy and applicability of the assessment or formulas. The specific factors help to tailor energy and nutrient recommendations for the individual. It is important to keep in mind that these assessments are only an estimate and should be considered a guide to tailor the next recommendations of the nutritional assessment. Key factors include:

1. Age—Equations that use an individual's age will be important because as we age there are changes in lean body mass and metabolic rate decreases with age.
2. Gender—It is important to utilize gender specific equations due to the differences in body composition between males and females. Body composition differences in genders can be found between muscle mass versus fat mass, and hormonal status or levels may influence needs.
3. Client weight history—A current weight and history of an individual will provide insight on weight trends or patterns that can be strongly correlated with health status. This also assesses risk for chronic conditions depending on either weight loss or weight gain.
4. Client height—An individual's height is the last essential factor that is needed in equations, as it is needed for calculating BMI and estimating energy needs.

Additional measures that are utilized in clinical and research areas will use the above in conjunction with the following:

1. Recumbent length—this measurement is in the field when collecting information on infants and young children (typically under the age of two who cannot stand on their own) to monitor growth. The World Health Organization will use the child's height and weight to plot on a chart to show growth overtime and can be a key indicator of the child's nutritional status.
2. Circumferences—this is a group of body girth measurements that will be taken at specific anatomical points to assess an individual's body composition, fat distribution, and potential health risks. In children, a crucial indicator of growth and brain growth, a head circumference will be utilized, and the Mid-Upper Arm Circumference (MUAC) indicates tissue growth. For all others, body circumference measure-

ments include waist, hip, arm, thigh, and calf. Circumference measurements are an inexpensive and simple way to assess individuals on the physical body and strongly relate measurements to increased risk for cardiovascular and metabolic disorders.

3. Limb lengths—measurements such as arm and leg length can be the entire length, limb segments, or projected lengths. To make these measurements, a practitioner will need to understand and find specific anatomical landmarks using a tape measure or calipers.
4. Sagittal abdominal diameter (SAD)—specifically quantifies visceral obesity or central fat around the abdominal region. There is a strong correlation between the measure of visceral obesity and predicting cardiovascular and metabolic risks in clinical practice.
5. Skinfold thickness—this type of measurement requires a tool called a caliper, otherwise known as the Lange caliper, to measure an individual's subcutaneous fat in various areas around the body. Once the skinfolds are measured, they are summed for a total and then put into an equation that accounts for gender, age, and in some equations, population, or ethnic specificity. The calculation will yield a body fat percentage (BF%) prediction for the individual and conceptualization of fatty tissue distribution throughout the body.

Finally, anthropometric indices are used to make inferences about body composition, growth, and development. The stacking of assessments with the indices improves predictive power and the ability to interpret the data more effectively.

1. Body Mass Index (BMI), or the Quetelet index—previously defined, can be used in clinical settings as well as a population screening tool to indicate an individual's weight status in relation to risk of chronic disease.
2. Waist-to-hip ratio (WHR)—this measurement falls under the body circumference measurements that are defined by the

waist circumference divided by the hip circumference. This method can be used for individual and population screening to indicate risk for health conditions. It should be noted that there are gender-specific ratio indicators: above 0.90 for males and above 0.85 for females [1].

3. Waist-to-height ratio (WHtR)—this measurement utilizes the circumference of the waist divided by individual's body height to measure the fat distribution. Higher values that are found correlate to obesity, central adiposity, and increased risk of cardiovascular disease. A reported value of over 0.5 indicates the increased risk for both genders, ages, and ethnic specific values.
4. Ponderal index (PI)—this is a similar measure to BMI; however, the equation differs: weight (grams) × 100/Length^3 (cm). If the result yields less than the 10th percentile, it will indicate malnutrition. This method is more appropriate for determining leanness or who is shorter or taller in nature.
5. Fat mass index (FMI)—is a potential indicator of an individual's body adiposity and can be useful in determining overall health. FMI is a ratio that uses fat mass in relation to height and considers age and gender regardless of lean mass. The use of dual x-ray absorptiometry (DEXA) scans has helped to provide precise analysis of body tissue components such as fat, muscle, and bone.
6. Fat-free mass index (FFMI)—another way to assess an individual's body composition to other individuals who have a similar body composition but differ in height. The index can calculate the amount of muscle mass relative to height.

The anthropometric measures rely on patient-specific factors to determine and evaluate the overall disease risk factors. Using the measures as standalone or combined assessments to evaluate disease risk will enhance the overall nutritional assessment. The last thing to consider is the advantages and disadvantages of anthropometry.

Advantages	Disadvantages
Measures can be objective with high specificity and sensitivity	User errors in measurements
Utilizing several measures or a combination can increase the significance of assessment	Differences in reference standards, domestic versus international standards
Readings are reproducible and can be compared to standard growth charts	Statistical cut-off levels for abnormal or normal levels can be arbitrary within populations
Inexpensive, easy to learn, and implement	Measurements reflect current status and not acute or chronic changes

Medical History An individual's medical history is important to evaluate as part of the assessment. Identifying nutrition-related conditions that reveal reasons for medications and supplements, along with weight loss or weight gain issues, can be crucial. Additionally, acute or chronic illnesses, existing medical conditions, and stressors can be added to equations to reflect metabolic demands or calorie needs. Examples of illnesses that can increase metabolic demands can include burns to the skin and body, cancers, auto-immune diseases, and metabolic disorders. Accounting for these conditions in medical history, we help to guide the individual's assessment.

Within medical history screening questions, additional emphasis should also focus on chronic health conditions. Clinical conditions can increase a patient's energy requirements. Chronic conditions may lead to increased or decreased calorie energy expenditure, which could increase the risk of nutrient malnutrition. An accurate assessment of resting metabolic rate (RMR) and estimated energy requirement (EER) should never be conducted without the consideration of all relevant conditions. Once the chronic health condition is accounted for, the anthropometric values will be used to determine an appropriate energy requirement and then effective nutritional support.

Clinical Assessment This part of the assessment will require a comprehensive and systemic investigation of physical signs and symptoms associated with malnutrition and deficiency of vitamins and minerals. Information that will be collected includes physical analysis of hair, nails, mouth, gums, eyes, tongue, bones, and thyroid gland. This information will help to detect the relevant signs that can help to establish an individual nutritional diagnosis.

Biochemical Data During clinical assessment, monitoring and objective information from biochemical testing can provide reliable measures of nutritional status. Examples could include hemoglobin levels to assess iron status; fasting blood glucose will measure current blood sugar levels, and albumin levels can evaluate protein status. To obtain these tests, a registered dietitian will work with an individual's medical team and physician to interpret the objective lab values along with the medical history. There are several common biochemical markers that help to determine the appropriate nutritional interventions and possible treatments. Specific lab tests could include:

- Analysis of hair, nails, and skin for deficiencies from micronutrients (vitamins and minerals) and protein status.
- Individual nutrient measurements in bodily fluids, such as urine and blood, can assess kidney function, signs of infection, and metabolic issues (glucose, ketones, and inflammation).
- Lipid profiles are collected through a blood panel that evaluates total cholesterol, low-density lipoprotein (LDL), high-density lipoprotein (HDL), and triglycerides.

Advantages	Disadvantages
Precise, accurate, and reproducible	Time consuming and expensive
Detect early changes in metabolism and nutrition before clinical manifestation occurs	Testing cannot be applied to large populations
Validates data acutely and chronically	Need assistance from trained personnel and facilities

Regular monitoring of individual biochemical markers will help health care providers to determine effective nutritional support and treatment if deficiencies or illness are found. These biochemical markers are essential to assess overall health status and can inform providers how the energy equations and therefore energy requirements can be interpreted and adjusted for the individual.

When evaluating a patient's nutritional and health status, it is essential to consider a comprehensive range of factors that directly influence energy requirements. Patient-specific elements such as age, sex, body composition, activity level, and metabolic conditions play a critical role in determining the accuracy of anthropometric measurements and the selection of appropriate energy equations. A thorough medical history provides insight into chronic diseases, medications, and inflammation that could skew or change weight-based calculations. Biochemical data will offer insight into metabolic stress or catabolic states that may necessitate adjustments to standard predictive equations. Integrating these variables ensures a more precise estimation of energy needs and supports individualized nutritional planning. Together, these components form a holistic picture that guides personalized care and effective nutritional planning.

Accuracy Limitations of Equations

Background There are approximately 138 known predictive equations to use to estimate an individual's metabolic and daily energy requirement. The predictive equations in large research and professional facilities have been debated on which equation is most appropriate for clients and/or patients. The equations provide a practical and non-invasive way to estimate energy needs and create personalized nutrition for individuals and specific populations that can include physical activity. In general, the formulas use large cohorts to establish reliability and validity for use; therefore, deciding which one is the best fit for an individual can be important. While not perfectly accurate for every individual or population, the equations offer a prediction or guideline that can be assimilated into the nutritional assessment and overall health outcomes.

Overestimation/Underestimation Some equations may over- or underestimate energy needs, particularly for individuals with specific medical conditions or unusual body composition. Patient-specific factors (sex, age, weight, and activity level) are a part of the equations and cannot account for an individual's metabolic differences. For example, an individual's metabolic rate can change significantly due to chronic conditions or being critically ill. These chronic conditions would not be factored into the equations and ultimately lead to an over- or under-prediction of energy needs. These types of limiting factors are methodological issues that can be difficult to control for. However, accounting for patient-specific and activity factors will help to guide individual results in larger populations. Here are some other considerations when discussing over- or underestimating energy needs:

1. Obese adults—The energy estimation equations can be problematic for obese patients due to the equations only considering the patient's established specific factors (age, gender, height, and weight). First, inaccuracies can be from the variations in body composition, for example, the differentiations between lean body mass and fat mass. In addition, an individual's metabolic imbalances and genetic factors are not accounted for in the traditional equations. More specifically, in this population, the equations fall short when compared to nonobese individuals in three areas. As noted above, there is an inadequate consideration for an individual's body composition. The standard estimation equations cannot distinguish between tissues; fat mass tends to be higher and can significantly influence caloric energy expenditure.

   Second, the energy estimation equations have had a high degree of individual physiological variability across the population, which can be pronounced in obese individuals. Higher amounts of fat mass are less metabolically active than lean tissue, which in turn will lower resting energy expenditure (REE). At rest, fat tissue burns fewer calories when compared to muscles at rest. Conversely, the total energy expenditure in some individuals may still be elevated due to the higher fat mass due to the overall body size that more overall tissue supports, moves, and regulates. For example, estimating basal metabolic rate (BMR) tends to be less accurate in obese individuals compared to those who are nonobese, with a noticeable increase in individual errors. Among the equations studied, the Mifflin-St Jeor equation performed the best, maintaining a relatively higher accuracy. It correctly predicted BMR in 70% of obese individuals, compared to 82% accuracy in nonobese adults. When errors occurred, underestimations were more common than overestimations. The largest discrepancy observed was a 20% underestimation and a 15% overestimation of measured BMR [2].

This will be discussed more when the individual equations are investigated; however, knowing the nuances between equations and specific populations will be pivotal. In the consideration of body composition, obese individuals' increased body mass is not proportionally predictable when compared to nonobese, as the equations often will overestimate or underestimate needs.

2. Limited accuracy in specific populations—The energy estimation equations inaccuracies can extend to specific populations who may not fit the healthy population definitions. Groups can include:
   - *Older adults*—the estimations are developed using data from younger adults and will not reflect the metabolic changes that are associated with aging. In research, it has been suggested that accuracy is low for patients over the age of 65 [3]. If an energy estimate is needed for an older individual, there are more specific equations that account for aging.
   - *Critically ill or hospitalized patients*—estimations for individuals in Intensive Care Units (ICUs) or other long-term clinical settings will need to account for metabolic changes, altered physiological states, and decreased physical activ-

ity. Illness and medical conditions significantly alter metabolism; for example, patients with cirrhosis experience a state of hypermetabolism due to inflammation or increased metabolic activity in the other organs. The estimation equation cannot account for this state and may underestimate the energy or caloric need.

- *Ethnic minorities*—original research that created the energy estimation equations primarily included white Europeans and Americans to establish the data and validity for use. However, using this specific population limits the ability to use the equation for general population usage. Studies have shown that common equations overestimate resting metabolic rate (RMR) [4], and it may be more prudent to use a combination of available equations that account for other factors that can account for ethnic variation in fat-free mass and metabolic rates [5].
- *Athletes and very active individuals*—energy estimation equations for this population will need to account for the physical activity levels (PAL) or needs/possible differences in lean body mass. PAL factors will use the intensity and duration of the specific activity to determine the estimate of energy or calories that will be used on top of baseline energy needs. In addition, athletes typically have a higher proportion of metabolic, lean body mass when compared to the general population. These considerations will be essential and should be used when available for the most accurate results. One example is the Cunningham equation; this preferred equation considers body composition/lean body mass (fat-free mass) as it provides a more accurate predictor of energy needs [6].

When considering and utilizing the energy estimation equations in nutritional assessment, it is essential to recognize the potential for both overestimation and underestimation, especially in populations with atypical body composition or clinical conditions. These inaccuracies can lead to inappropriate nutritional interventions, impacting patient outcomes, recovery, and long-term health. By understanding the limitations of predictive formulas and considering patient-specific factors such as fat mass, lean body mass, physical activity levels, and metabolic stress, clinicians can make more informed decisions.

Classification of Nutritional Status

The nutritional status of an individual can be important for identifying malnutrition or obesity, monitoring growth, body composition, and developing clinical interventions. This type of classification provides a non-invasive and cost-effective way to assess nutritional health. The core measurements or patient specifics of height, weight, waist circumference, and skinfolds can be the basis of information. The addition of the BMI and estimated energy equations will help to interpret how the data compares to established limits or critical cutoffs within a population. Individually, anthropometric measures and estimated energy equations are not as strong or powerful when they are used together as the combination of the two provides a complete picture. Using both methods then provides an objective assessment of tracking physical changes that can be made and a more reliable indication of an individual's energy balance. Two other vital reasons for combining the methods are the cause-and-effect relationship and the comprehensive risk analysis.

A cause-and-effect relationship can be defined by tracking the anthropometric changes by measuring BMI to note changes. For example, a low BMI indicates physical changes in weight (lower) which can signal a problem. The estimation of energy equations can help to identify and quantitatively estimate energy deficits or imbalances that led to changes in physical state. Comprehensive risk analysis uses the combined methods for a holistic understanding of an individual's health. Again, if we use the above example of an individual with a change weight that indicates a low BMI and then determine that there is a deficit of total calories, health providers can more accurately predict, diagnosis, classify and plan how to guide an individual's nutritional needs.

Chapter Summary

The use of the anthropometrics measures collects valuable and quantifiable data, not just numbers. The data collected will be a powerful indicator of health and potential health risks. Within a nutritional assessment, gathering of anthropometric data can evaluate an individual within a population or a larger population. In either case, focusing on overnutrition (obesity) or malnutrition (emaciation), ultimately data from the measures can assess overall and central fat body composition. The dual approach strengthens objectivity by pairing measurable physical changes with calculated estimates, reducing reliance on self-reported intake. Ultimately, combining both methods allows for a holistic evaluation of nutritional health, linking visible effects such as BMI changes with the energy imbalances that drive them, and supporting more precise risk analysis and intervention planning. Thoughtful consideration of the data can help transform the rest of the nutritional assessment and focus on individual-centered strategies.

Chapter Review Questions

1. Why might standard nutritional assessment equations under- or over-estimate energy needs in certain populations, and what factors contribute to these inaccuracies?
2. How do patient-specific characteristics such as age, sex, body composition, and metabolic conditions influence the selection and accuracy of energy estimation equations?
3. In what ways do anthropometric indices contribute to understanding body composition, growth, and development, and how does "stacking" assessments improve interpretation?
4. What advantages arise from combining multiple data points with the strengths of a chosen equation when making nutritional recommendations for an individual?

References

1. "Waist Circumference and Waist–Hip Ratio, Report of a WHO Expert Consultation". World Health Organization. 8–11 December 2008.
2. Frankenfield D, Roth-Yousey L, Compher C. Comparison of predictive equations for resting metabolic rate in healthy nonobese and obese adults: a systematic review. J Am Diet Assoc. 2005;105(5):775–89. https://doi.org/10.1016/j.jada.2005.02.005.
3. Porter J, Ward LC, Nguo K, Ward A, Davidson Z, Gibson S, Prentice R, Neuhouser ML, Truby H. Development and validation of age-specific predictive equations for total energy expenditure and physical activity levels for older adults. Am J Clin Nutr. 2024;119(5):1111–21. https://doi.org/10.1016/j.ajcnut.2024.02.005.
4. Miller S, Milliron BJ, Woolf K. Common prediction equations overestimate measured resting metabolic rate in young Hispanic women. Top Clin Nutr. 2013;28(2):120–35. https://doi.org/10.1097/TIN.0b013e31828d7a1b.
5. Reneau J, Obi B, Moosreiner A, et al. Do we need race-specific resting metabolic rate prediction equations? Nutr Diabetes. 2019;9:21. https://doi.org/10.1038/s41387-019-0087-8.
6. Thompson JT, Manore MM. Predicted and measured resting metabolic rate of male and female endurance athletes. J Am Diet Assoc. 96(1):30–4. ISSN 0002-8223. https://doi.org/10.1016/S0002-8223(96)00010-7.

Common Equations Used for Estimating Energy

4

Abstract

Accurate estimation of energy requirements is essential for effective nutritional assessment and intervention, particularly in diverse populations. This chapter explores the variability and limitations of commonly used predictive equations including Harris-Benedict, Mifflin-St. Jeor, Owen, Schofield (FAO/WHO/UNU), Henry Oxford, Katch-McArdle, and Cunningham. The information emphasizes the importance of selecting equations based on population-specific characteristics such as body composition, gender, and activity level. Additionally, it addresses the historical context and demographic limitations of foundational datasets, such as the Schofield database, and introduces the Henry Oxford equation as a more contemporary alternative. These insights support a more nuanced, individualized approach to energy estimation in clinical and performance nutrition settings.

Keywords

Basal metabolic rate (BMR) · Total daily energy expenditure (TDEE) · Predictive equations · Estimating calories · Physical activity · Resting metabolic rate (RMR) · Indirect calorimetry (IC)

S. Kitts, *Nutritional Assessment*,
https://doi.org/10.1007/978-3-032-22506-1_4

Learning Objectives
By the end of this chapter students should be able to:

- Describe the purpose, structure, and historical development of major predictive energy equations, including Harris-Benedict, Mifflin-St. Jeor, Owen, Schofield, Henry Oxford, Katch-McArdle, and Cunningham.
- Explain the population-specific characteristics—such as body composition, gender, age, and activity level—that influence the accuracy and applicability of energy estimation equations.
- Analyze the limitations of foundational datasets (e.g., the Schofield database) and evaluate how these limitations affect equation validity in diverse populations.
- Compare the strengths, weaknesses, and practical considerations of commonly used predictive equations in clinical and performance nutrition settings.

The time has come to put knowledge into practice as this chapter will explore common equations that are used to estimate energy individuals' basal metabolic and total energy requirements. As previously discussed, there are hundreds of such equations that could be used; however, researchers and organizations have found the most appropriate equations based on population specifics. The equations have a range of considerations such as ethnicity, activity levels, body composition, and age. Use of the wrong equation may lead to over- or underestimation of energy needs, which can be a large misstep in the assessment of an individual that affects the overall recommendations.

Each equation that is discussed will provide background information, population specificity or considerations, validity in practice, and limitations. The importance of including these pieces will help practitioners decide the most appropriate equation to use for an individual. Additionally, practitioner comfortability and knowledge of one to two equations they can rely on use improves the quality of the assessment and future recommendations. It should be noted that the equations that are discussed in this chapter use the most common variation of the formula. There is no single equation that can capture or perfectly determine the energy expenditure for every individual or health parameter. The different equations that have been developed were created and validated based on a need to study a certain population. The inevitable trade-offs for each equation toggle between accuracy, practicality, availability, and need. Even with populations with shared characteristics, there is a possibility the equation may be more accurate for one part of a population and less accurate for another. One other consideration for equations of validity and reliability is time. Some of the equations were developed over a hundred years ago, and as researchers gain more data and insight, there will be a need to update the equations. Minor adjustments in the constants of the equations may change to reflect changes in population characteristics.

Furthermore, this chapter will show examples of the equation process. To ensure a seamless learning process, a data block will be provided that will be utilized for each equation. A data block will give the gender, age, height, weight, and any other pertinent information that will be used in each equation. Through years of trial and error, having a set data block of information can show the variances of the equations and the reach of their use.

Components of the Equations

A quick review of the necessary components of each of the equations will be provided. The importance of these items will increase the accuracy and individuality of the data for the individual. Please note that the units that are more commonly used in energy equations will be weight in kilograms (kg) and height in meters (m). These units are part of the International System of Units (SI), which offers a global standard in research and data collection for the ease of collaboration and understanding of results.

Weight (kg) is a key component of nutritional assessment that can indicate overall nutritional status. Weight is an indicator of changes in the body's energy and nutrient stores, which can be crucial during nutritional assessment. Additionally, weight can be combined with height to calculate Body Mass Index (BMI), determine energy and macronutrient baselines versus activity needs, and monitor weight changes over time. Converting weight from pounds to kilograms will require dividing pounds by 2.2.

Height (m/cm) is used in nutritional assessment as a key indicator of long-term health through critical growth periods. Specifically in children, it reflects growth overtime and is used to identify malnutrition or stunted growth. Use of standardized growth charts shows height and weight in terms of percentiles when compared to peers. In adults, height can be an indicator of long-term health and standard of living. This indicator can be described as a product of cumulative nutrition and activity for an adult's lifespan. Converting height in inches to meters will require multiplying inches by 0.0254. When you calculate the meters, be sure to also determine meters squared (m^2) and centimeters (cm) as these values will be used in different equations.

Age is another key factor regarding nutritional assessment, as age significantly impacts an individual's dietary requirements. Most nutritional recommendations should be adjusted based on a person's age because the relationship between age and energy need is not linear. This means that as we age, the energy required to maintain daily energy functions does decrease. This is due to the natural losses in muscle or lean body mass, which in turn decrease the amount of metabolically active tissue.

Gender is a crucial component in energy equations and the nutritional assessment and is used to educate or modify nutritional recommendations based on definite physiological differences between males and females. Males biologically have a higher percentage of total lean muscle mass and lower percentage of body fat when compared to females that are same age and weight. Due to the higher percentage of lean muscle mass in males, the tissue is more metabolically active, which will require more energy to maintain daily energy functions. There are formulas in this chapter that will adjust the gender differences in body composition and metabolism to provide more accurate estimates.

Data Block (for the Chapter)

Gender	Female	Additional information and conversions
Age	42	
Height	5′6″	66 in/1.67 m/2.82 m^2/167.64 cm
Weight	180	81.82 kg
Physical activity level (PAL)	1.6	She has been trying to lose weight over the past 6 months. Physical activity is 5 days/wk, 30–35 min of moderate intensity
% Body fat	36%	Measured by calipers method

Equations Used for Basal Metabolic Rate and Total Daily Energy Expenditure

Harris-Benedict Equation

Background Information F.G. Benedict and J.A. Harris published the prediction equation in the early twentieth century to determine human basal metabolism as a part of several studies. The purpose of these first prediction equations was to be used as benchmark to establish normal standards to compare individuals for clinical and research purposes [1]. These equations are commonly still used in clinical settings to estimate an individual's basal metabolic rate (BMR), which can help to determine caloric needs for weight management and assess energy requirements of those individuals with disease states.

This equation does account for gender differences as the formula includes separate values for men and women which acknowledges physiological differences in energy expenditures. More specifically, the formulas contain different values and coefficients used for weight, height, and age, reflecting the known differences in body composition and metabolism values between males and females.

The equation involves two steps to ultimately estimate total daily energy expenditure (TDEE): first calculating the BMR and then applying an activity multiplier that corresponds to set values of typical activity levels. The physical activity levels (PAL) are highlighted below [2]:

There have been several revisions and evolutions to the original Harris-Benedict equation that have improved the correlation of the coefficients for both genders and simplified the equation. The revisions increased the sample sizes and utilized a wider age range to improve reliability and validity [3].

Population The original Harris-Benedict prediction equation was based on 239 subjects with an age range of participants of 21–70 years [3]. Initially, the prediction equation was developed for healthy, normal weight individuals to establish baseline standards. This will be a consideration for practitioners to consider when choosing this equation.

Validity and Limitations This prediction equation is seen as moderately valid, showing that it can overestimate energy needs in certain individuals, specifically those who are overweight or obese. It also may not be accurate for those who have different activity levels based on the rest of the population, such as the elderly and individuals with acute or chronic diseases [4]. Other reasons for limited validity could include outdated data, population-specific or ethnicity accuracy, and body composition variances.

Therefore, Harris-Benedict should be used as a starting point to determine BMR and TDEE. Adjusting for individual patient-specific values and circumstances will need to be considered or the use of a more modern equation.

Equation

(Males) BMR = 66.4730 + (13.7516 × weight in kg) + (5.0033 × height in cm) – (6.7550 × age in years)

(Females) BMR = 655.0955 + (9.5634 × weight in kg) + (1.8496 × height in cm) – (4.6756 × age in years)

Example: (Female)
BMR = 655.0955 + (9.5634 × weight in kg) + (1.8496 × height in cm) - (4.6756 × age in years)
BMR = 655.0955 + (9.5634 × 81.82 kg) + (1.8496 × 167.6 4 cm) - (4.6756 × 42)
BMR = 655.0955 + (782.477) + (310.067)–(196.375)
BMR = 1551.26 calories
TDEE = BMR × PAL (activity level)
TDEE = 1551.26 × 1.6
TDEE = 2482.02 calories

Mifflin-St. Jeor Equation

Background In 1990, MD Mifflin and ST St. Jeor published the revised Harris-Benedict equation and improved estimation resting metabolic rate (RMR) to include both obese and non-obese individuals. The improvements to the equation came from the inclusion of indirect calorimetry and a multiple regression analysis of the data [5].

Indirect calorimetry (IC) is used to measure the exact calorie requirements via a mask or hood to collect exhaled gases. Once the gases are collected, they are analyzed to determine the oxygen consumption and carbon dioxide production as this is proportional to the amount of energy being produced. The correlation can be physiologically explained by the body breaking down the macronutrients through digestion that creates heat, carbon dioxide, and water. Therefore, the amount of expelled carbon dioxide produced is proportional to the amount of energy an individual uses. Mifflin and St. Jeor used the IC measurement to develop their predictive equation to improve the accuracy and to service a more diverse population of healthy individuals.

Table 4.1 Physical Activity Levels designations to needed to find TDEE

Sedentary (little to no exercise)	BMR × 1.2
Lightly active (light exercise 1–3 days/week)	BMR × 1.375
Moderately active (moderate exercise 3–5 days/week)	BMR × 1.55
Very active (hard exercise 6–7 days/week)	BMR × 1.725
Extra active (very hard, physical job, or training twice a day)	BMR × 1.9

The main part of the equation is the same for both genders; however, there is gender-specific constant added at the end (+5 for men, −161 for women). Additionally, this equation will be a two-step process; calculation of RMR followed by multiplying a PAL factor that corresponds to daily activity level. The same PAL designation will be used as the previous equation, referring to Table 4.1 to find the appropriate multiplier.

Population The work to improve the equations 'validity included 498 subjects with an age range of participants of 19–78 [5]. Additionally, the sample inclusion of different body composition types (obese and non-obese) increases the use of the equation in clinical and health settings where direct measurements such as whole room calorimetry are not possible. There is some evidence for this equation to perform well for females across different weight statuses (healthy, overweight, and obese), and it is preferred for adults of different body compositions [6].

Validity and Limitations This equation is currently the most accurate for calculating RMR in individuals with normal BMI (i.e., with the index between 19 and 25) when it is not necessary to know the percentage of body fat. This prediction equation predicts resting metabolic rate at 10% of that measured by indirect calorimetry in more non-obese and obese subjects, is higher than any other equation, and has the lowest error rate [7]. However, there are noted situations where the prediction equation might be less suitable for certain populations: athletes [8], children and adolescents [9], and individuals with multiple comorbidities [10].

The Mifflin St. Jeor is regarded as one of the most accurate formulas for predicting resting metabolic energy needs for the general population. The inclusion of IC to predict calorie expenditure by Mifflin St. Jeor improves the previous equation, broadening the application in various settings. Although it is not precise for every individual (unique body composition or specific health conditions), it can serve as a broad-reaching equation that will give systematic and individualized calorie expenditure.

Equation

(Males) RMR = (10 × weight in kg) + (6.25 × height in cm) – (5 × age in years) + 5

(Females) RMR = (10 × weight in kg) + (6.25 × height in cm) – (5 × age in years) – 161

Example: (Female)

RMR = (10 × weight in kg) + (6.25 × height in cm) – (5 × age in years) – 161

RMR = (10 × 81.82 kg) + (6.25 × 167.64 cm) – (5 × 42) – 161

RMR = (818.20) + (1047.75) – (210) – 161

RMR = 1494.95 calories

TDEE = RMR × PAL (activity level)

TDEE = 1494.95 × 1.6

TDEE = 2391.92 calories

Henry Oxford equation

Background J. Henry and international collaborators gathered a global dataset between 1995 and 2005. Investigating the predictive equations, Henry identified that other equations failed to account for the ethnic body composition variations. Earlier data sets were integrated with the researcher's inclusions and then analyzed with a mathematical regression to develop the more inclusive equation. Due to the size of the data set, it yielded the development of the "Henry" equations and the "Oxford" database to improve BMR predictions of energy equations.

The expansion of the database and equations had several impacts on assessing nutrition globally. Improved accuracy for underrepresented populations, increased use in clinical assessment of populations at-risk, and helped public health professionals to establish more recommendations or guidelines for energy intake. The diversity of the data set could be its strongest asset.

Population The collaboration developed a database that housed 10,552 RMR values from a diverse population that included 5794 males and 4702 females from both developed and developing countries [11]. The data set adjusted some of the ethnic groups by excluding all subjects of Italian descent due to an oversaturation in other data sets and included subjects from tropical regions to increase the ethnicity and global reach of the equation.

Validity and Limitations Improved accuracy by expanding the data set to include a more diverse population is noted. Studies do show a strong correlation between the predicted RMR equations and actual RMR, which can indicate predictive accuracy [12]. However, limitations begin with how the data set has aged. There have not been any updates since the original data collection and development of the equations. A contemporary refresh of the data set that would assess modern populations' changes. Additionally, the equations have been criticized for the assumption of a linear relationship between RMR and individuals' reported body weight [11]. As individuals age, there are increases in general weight, non-lean mass, and RMR decreases. This association would then indicate that the equation may not be appropriate for overweight and older populations.

The Henry Oxford equations provide a method for estimating energy in a broader inclusion of underrepresented groups. The gender-specific equations are further assessed by age ranges that will use body composition data to predict metabolic rates. There is no activity factor or PAL that is applied after finding the RMR.

Equation

Sex	Age	Oxford/Henry BMR Equation (Metric)
Males	18–30	BMR = 14.4 × Body Mass + 3.13 × Height + 113
	30–60	BMR = 11.4 × Body Mass + 5.41 × Height – 137
	60+	BMR = 11.4 × Body Mass + 5.41 × Height – 256
Females	18–30	BMR = 10.4 × Body Mass + 6.15 × Height – 282
	30–60	BMR = 8.18 × Body Mass + 5.02 × Height – 11.6
	60+	BMR = 8.52 × Body Mass + 4.21 × Height + 10.7

Mass in kilograms, height in centimeters

Example: (Female 30–60)
BMR = 8.18 × Body Mass + 5.02 × Height – 11.6
BMR = 8.18 × 81.82 + 5.02 × 167.64 – 11.6
BMR = 1499.24 calories

Owen Equation

Background Owen and colleagues developed this equation in the 1980s to estimate RMR/REE, relying on individual body weight alone. In developing this equation, the researchers used a small sample size and strictly regulated the investigation as participants were admitted to a research center [13]. The researchers identified the mathematical relationship between subjects' measured IC and reported body weight. By doing this, the equation is simplified and decreased by the other patient with specific reported variables. Initially the data set was female-centric, 1986–1987 then expanded the equation to include both genders. Additionally, from the 1987 study on females, it yielded a separate equation specifically for female athletes: RMR = 50.4 + 21.1 × weight (in kg) [13]. It should be noted that this Owen athletic formula is less common than other athletic-specific equations and is not widely used or cited in research often.

This equation for predicting resting energy is a simpler alternative to other equations. The use of only body weight for the individual makes the equation a practical tool that estimates resting energy and can easily be interpreted for educational purposes. For specific populations where weight or weight changes would be the dominant variable, this equation may be a good alternative, as other variables such as height, weight, and age would not be needed [14].

Population The researchers recruited forty-four females with a mixed body composition, lean to obese, whose ages ranged from 18 to 65 [13]. Within the forty-four subjects, eight were identified as trained athletes (lean body composition and measured IC values), and the other participants were found to have mixed body compositions (lean to obese). It was determined that this equation could be utilized in healthy, non-athletic populations. A male-specific equation was added after the initial female study by using IC and determining the constant variables that would be used in addition to body weight.

Validity and Limitations The Owen equation delivers a quick estimate and relies on its simplistic prediction for resting energy requirements. The overall reported validity for the Owen equation is mixed and dependent on the population being studied. The varying accuracy between groups can be seen with specific examples such as sedentary middle-aged adults with obesity reporting the most accuracy and severely underestimating RMR in adults with various disease states. Ultimately, the Owen equation will provide more reliable accuracy in estimating REE for groups rather than an individual assessment.

A large limitation to the equations is the elimination of age, height, weight, or any other underlying conditions into consideration, so the final calculation is only an estimate of the patients' REE caloric total. Since the introduction of the formula, the accuracy of equation has been shown to incorrectly estimate the energy requirements for females and males. In specific populations such as females that have lost weight or are utilizing calorie-restricted diets, it may be a useful predictor of resting energy [14]. Additionally, the development and improvement of more complex formulas eclipsed the Owen formula as the inclusion of other patient-specific factors were included.

The Owen equation provides an estimate of resting energy and should be paired with other factors that would improve accuracy. If practitioners would use this equation, understanding the over- or underestimation of REE in populations outside of the original targeted healthy, normal weight adults, it can be used as a quick rough estimate. The need for a quick assessment should not outweigh the benefit of accurate assessment for a more individual approach.

Equation

MALES: REE = 879 + 10.2 (weight in kg)
FEMALES: REE = 795 + 7.2 (weight in kg)

Example:
REE = 795 + 7.2 (weight in kg)
REE = 795 + 7.2 (81.82)
REE = 795 + 589.10
REE = 1384.10 calories

Schofield and FAO/WHO/UNU

Background The Schofield equations were designed by W. Schofield in the 1980s to estimate basal metabolic rate (BMR) in adults and children. Formulas were derived from a large dataset that included pediatric and adult subject information. The dataset population included Europeans (mainly Italian), Americans, and Asians subjects that also encompassed developed and underdeveloped countries [15]. The equations are different from the previous equations discussed, as there are different formulas based on gender and age and have an expanded section for injury factors (IF) and activity factors.

In 1985, the Schofield equations were incorporated into the FAO/WHO/UNU report to discuss the human energy requirements globally. The FAO/WHO/UNU utilized the Schofield database and refined the data utilizing a factorial method by summing the energy costs of occupational and nonoccupational activities and sleeping to determine the total energy expenditure [16]. The refinement of the Schofield data included more studies and data points, offering a broader range of population that ultimately improved the predictive power of the REE. Moving forward, the comprehensive set of equations is interchangeable or noted as "Schofield equations" recommended by FAO/WHO/UNU [16]. There was a revision in 2004 that incorporated newer data and improved accuracy in determining estimates for total energy expenditure (TEE).

Population Historically, the equations were initially based on datasets from developed countries in Western Europe and North America. The refinement of the datasets (over 7000 subjects from 23 countries) utilized international collaboration to achieve better global applicability and evaluate populations. This broader range can determine estimated energy requirements for all age groups, genders, and ethnic groups/populations, creating a common way to discuss estimated energy.

Validity and Limitations First, the overall validity of the Schofield equation varies significantly depending on the population being investigated. In 2018 there was a reanalysis of the equation, and it highlighted REE overestimation (approximately 8%) in all age groups overall and possibly higher in adults [17]. Second, the Schofield equations recommended by FAO/WHO/UNU are utilized for general use, and they have developed population-specific equations to provide more accurate estimates for geographical regions where the original data and equations could not be applied.

The Schofield-FAO/WHO/UNU equation is a widely used predictive formula for estimating basal metabolic rate (BMR), which represents the amount of energy expended by the body at rest to maintain vital physiological functions. It can serve as a foundational tool in nutritional assessment and clinical evaluation for determining daily energy requirements. Despite its broad application, the equation has faced some criticism for limited population diversity in its original dataset, prompting the redevelopment and refinement to improve global considerations within populations. Moreover, the collaboration of these equations can assess and provide international recommendations for energy needs.

Equation(s)

FAO/WHO/UNU	Men	Age 10–18	: (16.6 × W in kg) + (77 × H in meter) + 572
		Age 18–30	: (15.4 × W in kg) − (27 × H in meter) + 717
		Age 30–60	: (11.3 × W in kg) + (16 × H in meter) + 901
		Age > 60	: (8.8 × W in kg) + (1128 × H in meter) − 1071
	Women	Age 10–18	: (7.4 × W in kg) + (482 × H in meter) + 217
		Age 18–30	: (13.3 × W in kg) + (334 × H in meter) + 35
		Age 30–60	: (8.7 × W in kg) − (25 × H in meter) + 865
		Age > 60	: (9.2 × W in kg) + (637 × H in meter) − 302

Example: Age 30–60
BMR = (8.7 × W in kg) − (25 × H in meter) + 865
BMR = (8.7 × 81.82 kg) − (25 × 1.68 m) + 865
BMR = (711.83)–(42) + 865
BMR = 1534.83 calories

Katch-McArdle

Background F. Katch and W. McArdle recruited 136 college males and females to participate in a study to evaluate the validity of body composition equations by utilizing hydrostatic weighing. Based on Archimedes' Principle of Displacement, the participant is submerged under water, and body density can be measured as fat tissue is lighter and muscle and bone heavier, which displaces the water. The measured value was then compared to prediction equations, and it was found that the equation could be useful in calculating BMR in healthy young adult subjects when you have access to lean body mass (LBM) values [18]. This equation is unique because it does consider an individual's LBM in addition to weight, height, weight, age, and gender.

As discussed previously, muscle tissues are more metabolically active when compared to fat tissues. An individual's LBM is a better indicator of their metabolic rate rather than total body weight. The Katch-McArdle equation will need the LBM percentage, or it will have to be calculated first. Once the LBM is determined, the value can be entered into the BMR equation. Finally. An activity level or PAL can be entered to find a total energy estimate (TEE).

Population For this equation, the population becomes very specific as it is indicated for individuals who exercise or are athletes, range in age of 17–24 years old, and have higher LBM values. The equation does not differentiate between gender and ethnicity. The equations of reliance on the LBM value and other factors such as age, gender, and medical conditions are less impactful and will make the equation less accurate in individuals with varying body compositions (overweight or obese) and advanced age.

Validity and Limitations The Katch-McArdle equation's validity is affected by age, followed by the percentage of LBM. Obtaining a true body fat percentage can be difficult as assessment tools such as underwater weighing, skin calipers, air displacement measures such as a BodPod, or dual-energy X-ray absorptiometry (DEXA) scans may not be available or cost-effective. However, if a percentage of body fat (%BF) can be obtained, the LBM can be calculated to find BMR and TEE.

The limitations of this equation become very clear based on the specific population. The equation therefore will not be suited for obese individuals due to higher fat percentages, older individuals even if they have a higher LBM, and individuals with medical conditions. Age-related metabolic changes or chronic health conditions influence metabolic rates and cannot be accounted for in this predictive equation.

While the Katch-McArdle equation offers a valuable tool for estimating metabolic rates, particularly for athletes and healthy young adults with known body composition, it has notable limitations when applied to individuals with atypical body types. Accurate body fat assessment is critical, and individual variability further complicates its reliability. Ultimately, this equation should be used as a flexible estimate rather than a definitive measure, with ongoing adjustments based on personal outcomes and individuals' training or physical activity needs.

Equation

1. Calculate Fat Mass: Fat Mass (in kg) = Total Body Weight (kg) × (Body Fat Percentage/100)
2. Calculate Lean Body Mass: Lean Body Mass (in kg) = Total Body Weight (kg) – Fat Mass (in kg).
3. BMR = 370 + (21.6 × lean body mass (kg))

Example:
FM = Total Body Weight (kg) × (Body Fat Percentage/100)
FM = 81.82 kg × (36%/100)
FM = 81.82 kg × .36 = 29.45 kg
LBM = Total Body Weight (kg) – Fat Mass (in kg)
LBM = 81.82 kg – 29.45 kg = 52.37 kg
BMR = 370 + (21.6 × lean body mass (kg))
BMR = 370 + (21.6 × 52.37 kg)
BMR = 370 + (1.130.98)
BMR = 1500.98 calories
*Option to calculate TEE
TEE = 1.6 PAL × 1500.98 calories
TEE = 2401.57 calories

Cunningham Equation

Background In 1980, J. Cunningham examined the factors that can influence BMR and the most significant factor. Through the study it was concluded that age, gender, physical activity, and body composition have an influence; however, the LBM factor was a significant factor in predicting resting energy in healthy individuals. Cunningham utilized select participants from the Harris-Benedict study to use LBM as the primary predictor in determining resting energy needs. In 1991, Cunningham reexamined the equation to improve accuracy by lowering the constant variables in the equation to reflect updated data. This in turn yielded a more conservative estimate of RMR for a larger population [19]. This equation, much like the Harris-Benedict, will need to have access to an individual's LBM to then determine the prediction of metabolic rate.

Population The original intent of this equation was its use in a general population; the use of LBM as part of the equation suggests it may be better suited for athletes (recreational or trained) [20]. The use of this formula has direct applications to sports nutrition and clinical settings when estimating energy needs in active populations. A more conservative estimate of RMR can provide valid information and education about calories needed to support activity and decrease the risk of overfeeding.

Validity and Limitations When using the Cunningham equation with an athletic population, the equation is the most accurate to predict RMR due largely to its use of LBM or fat free mass (FFM) [21]. For practitioners, knowing that this formula will be advantageous to use with an athletic population in conjunction with the availability of obtaining LBM measures more readily will benefit the individual's prediction for energy needs.

Limitations for the Cunningham equation can be identified through population variances. The 1980 equation, which is still used in some clinical settings, displayed an overestimation for RMR in populations with lower metabolic activity or altered physiology such as sedentary lifestyle or chronic disease states [19]. The revised 1991 equation has been cited as underestimating RMR in highly active or muscular individuals [22]. The slight over- and underestimation tendencies of this equation are well documented and will need to be carefully utilized in populations that fall outside the indicated population's use.

The Cunningham 1980 and 1991 equations both estimate the RMR and utilize the LBM or FFM as a key variable as age, gender, and height are eliminated from the equation. In education or clinical practice, the choice between these equations should be guided by the individual's body composition, physical activity level, and dietary goals.

Equation (LBM will need to be determined first & at end multiply by PAL at end to determine TEE)

Cunningham 1980 $RMR = 500 + 22 \times FFM$
Cunningham 1991 $RMR = 370 + 21.6 \times FFM$

Example: (1991 equation)
FM = Total Body Weight (kg) × (Body Fat Percentage/100)
FM = 81.82 kg × (36%/100)
FM = 81.82 kg × .36 = 29.45 kg
LBM = Total Body Weight (kg) – Fat Mass (in kg)
LBM = 81.82 kg – 29.45 kg = 52.37 kg
RMR = 370 + 21.6 × FFM
RMR = 370 + 21.6 × 52.37
RMR = 1501.19 calories
TEE = 1.6 × 1501.19
TEE = 2401.91 calories

Chapter Summary

Choosing a prediction energy equation that reflects the physical and demographic characteristics of the target population, such as gender, age, health status, and physical activity level, is essential for accurate energy assessment. While the Cunningham and Katch-McArdle equations were developed using general population data, it outperformed other models in recreational athletes, highlighting fat-free mass (FFM) as a key predictor of resting energy expenditure (REE). In contrast, FFM-based equations from Mifflin-St. Jeor and Owen, derived from lean and obese individuals, were less accurate in athletic populations. This suggests that body composition differences significantly influence equation performance.

The Henry Oxford equation, developed as an update to the Schofield equations, incorporates more recent and diverse data and may offer improved accuracy in certain populations. However, like other generalized models, its applicability to athletic or clinical groups should be evaluated carefully.

Additionally, caution is advised when using the ratio of measured to predicted RMR as a proxy for energy availability, especially from a single measurement. Historical databases like Schofield's, which informed the Schofield-FAO/WHO/UNU equations, included a disproportionate number of Italian participants, potentially limiting their applicability across diverse racial and ethnic groups.

Interpreting Variations Between Prediction Equations

The chart below highlights how different predictive equations yield varying estimates for resting energy expenditure (REE) and total daily energy expenditure (TDEE), even when applied to the same individual profile. These differences stem from the variables each equation prioritizes, such as weight, height, age, gender, and fat-free mass, and the populations they were originally developed from. As described in this chapter, some of the equations might not be appropriate for the example individual used for the chapter based on variables and purpose of the equation. Keeping this in mind, this chapter utilizes one individual's patient-specific characteristics for a uniform presentation of how the equations would yield the answers for energy prediction.

Equation	Resting energy estimate (BMR, RMR, REE)	Total energy estimate (TDEE, TEE)
Harris Benedict	1,551.26 calories	2,482.02 calories
Mifflin-St. Jeor	1,494.95 calories	2,391.92 calories
Henry Oxford	1,499.24 calories	
Owen	1,384.10 calories	
Schofield FAO/WHO/UNU	1,534.83 calories	2,455.73 calories
Katch-McArdle	1,500.98 calories	2,401.57 calories
Cunningham	1,501.19 calories	2,401.91 calories

Key anecdotal observations can be made:

- Harris-Benedict and Schofield FAO/WHO/UNU provide some of the highest estimates for both REE and TDEE, which may reflect their older datasets and broader population assumptions.

- Mifflin-St. Jeor, often considered more accurate for modern clinical use, gives a lower REE and TDEE than Harris-Benedict, suggesting a more conservative approach.
- Owen produces the lowest REE estimate, which may risk underfeeding if used without clinical context—especially in active or muscular individuals.
- Henry Oxford offers a REE like Mifflin and Cunningham but lacks a TDEE value in this comparison, limiting direct interpretation. These equations are mostly used to find resting metabolic values.
- Katch-McArdle and Cunningham, both based on fat-free mass, yield nearly identical REE and TDEE values, reinforcing the importance of body composition in energy prediction for athletic or lean populations.

These differences matter because it can help practitioners plan and execute the equations for that individual specifically and tailor the nutritional assessment. Moreover, considering the differences between the equations could help to minimize over- or underestimation of calories needed for the individual. For example, a difference of 100–200 calories per day can significantly impact nutritional planning, especially in clinical, athletic, or weight management settings. Overestimation may lead to unintended weight gain, while underestimation can result in inadequate energy intake and compromised recovery or performance. Selecting the most appropriate equation requires considering the individual's body composition, specific patient factors, physical activity level, and health status, not just convenience or ease of an equation.

In summary, no single equation is universally accurate. Selecting the most appropriate model requires understanding the population it was designed for and considering individual characteristics like age, body composition with variances for excess weight versus LBM, and physical activity level. Combining predictive equations with clinical judgment and direct measurements, if available, offers the most reliable approach to nutritional assessment.

Chapter Review Questions

1. Why is accurate estimation of energy requirements essential for effective nutritional assessment, and what challenges arise when applying predictive equations to diverse populations?
2. How do the Harris-Benedict, Mifflin-St. Jeor, and Henry Oxford equations differ in terms of their historical development, datasets, and population applicability?
3. Given a patient with atypical body composition (e.g., high lean mass, obesity, or sarcopenia), which predictive equations might be more appropriate, and why?
4. How does practitioner familiarity and comfort with specific equations influence the quality of nutritional assessments and subsequent recommendations?

References

1. Frankenfield DC, Muth ER, Rowe WA. The Harris-Benedict studies of human basal metabolism: history and limitations. J Am Diet Assoc [Internet]. 1998;98(4):439–45. Available from: https://doi.org/10.1016/S0002-8223(98)00100-X.
2. Harris JA, Benedict FG. A biometric study of human basal metabolism. Proc Natl Acad Sci USA. 1918;4(12):370–3.
3. Pavlidou E, Papadopoulou SK, Seroglou K, Giaginis C. Revised Harris–Benedict equation: new human resting metabolic rate equation. Metabolites. 2023;13(2):189. https://doi.org/10.3390/metabo13020189.
4. Bendavid I, Lobo DN, Barazzoni R, Cederholm T, Coëffier M, de van der Schueren M, et al. The centenary of the Harris-Benedict equations: how to assess energy requirements best? Recommendations from the ESPEN expert group. Clin Nutr [Internet]. 2021;40(3):690–701. Available from: https://doi.org/10.1016/j.clnu.2020.11.012.
5. Mifflin MD, St Jeor ST, Hill LA, Scott BJ, Daugherty SA, Koh YO. A new predictive equation for resting energy expenditure in healthy individuals. Am J Clin Nutr. 1990;51(2):241–7. https://doi.org/10.1093/ajcn/51.2.241.
6. Thom G, Gerasimidis K, Rizou E, et al. Validity of predictive equations to estimate RMR in females with varying BMI. J Nutr Sci. 2020;9:e17. Published 2020 May 26. https://doi.org/10.1017/jns.2020.11.
7. Frankenfield D, Roth-Yousey L, Compher C. Comparison of predictive equations for resting metabolic rate in healthy nonobese and obese adults: a systematic review. J Am Diet Assoc [Internet]. 2005;105(5):775–89. Available from: https://doi.org/10.1016/j.jada.2005.02.005.

8. O'Neill JER, Corish CA, Horner K. Accuracy of resting metabolic rate prediction equations in athletes: A systematic review with meta-analysis. Sports Med [Internet]. 2023;53(12):2373–98. Available from: https://doi.org/10.1007/s40279-023-01896-z.
9. Psota T, Chen KY. Measuring energy expenditure in clinical populations: rewards and challenges. Eur J Clin Nutr [Internet]. 2013;67(5):436–42. Available from: https://doi.org/10.1038/ejcn.2013.38.
10. Cancello R, Soranna D, Brunani A, Scacchi M, Tagliaferri A, Mai S, et al. Analysis of predictive equations for estimating resting energy expenditure in a large cohort of morbidly obese patients. Front Endocrinol (Lausanne) [Internet]. 2018;9:367. Available from: https://doi.org/10.3389/fendo.2018.00367.
11. Henry CJK. Basal metabolic rate studies in humans: measurement and development of new equations. Public Health Nutr [Internet]. 2005;8(7A):1133–52. Available from: https://doi.org/10.1079/phn2005801.
12. Galgani JE, Castro-Sepulveda M, Pérez-Luco C, Fernández-Verdejo R. Validity of predictive equations for resting metabolic rate in healthy humans. Clin Sci (Lond) [Internet]. 2018;132(16):1741–51. Available from: https://doi.org/10.1042/CS20180317.
13. Owen OE, Kavle E, Owen RS, Polansky M, Caprio S, Mozzoli MA, et al. A reappraisal of caloric requirements in healthy women. Am J Clin Nutr [Internet]. 1986;44(1):1–19. Available from: https://doi.org/10.1093/ajcn/44.1.1.
14. Almajwal AM, Abulmeaty MMA. New predictive equations for resting energy expenditure in normal to overweight and obese population. Int J Endocrinol [Internet]. 2019;2019:5727496. Available from: https://doi.org/10.1155/2019/5727496.
15. Fuentes-Servín J, Avila-Nava A, González-Salazar LE, Pérez-González OA, Servín-Rodas MDC, Serralde-Zuñiga AE, et al. Resting energy expenditure prediction equations in the pediatric population: a systematic review. Front Pediatr [Internet]. 2021;9:795364. Available from: https://doi.org/10.3389/fped.2021.795364.
16. National Academies of Sciences, Engineering, Medicine, Health, Medicine Division, Food, Nutrition Board, et al. Development of prediction equations for estimated energy requirements. Washington, DC: National Academies Press; 2023.
17. Wahrlich V, Teixeira TM, Anjos LAD. Validity of a population-specific BMR predictive equation for adults from an urban tropical setting. Clin Nutr [Internet]. 2018;37(1):208–13. Available from: https://doi.org/10.1016/j.clnu.2016.12.005.
18. Katch FI, McArdle WD. Validity of body composition prediction equations for college men and women. Am J Clin Nutr [Internet]. 1975;28(2):105–9. Available from: https://doi.org/10.1093/ajcn/28.2.105.

19. Miller S, Milliron B-J, Woolf K. Common prediction equations overestimate measured resting metabolic rate in young Hispanic women. Top Clin Nutr [Internet]. 2013;28(2):120–35. Available from: https://doi.org/10.1097/TIN.0b013e31828d7a1b.
20. ten Haaf T, Weijs PJM. Resting energy expenditure prediction in recreational athletes of 18–35 years: confirmation of Cunningham equation and an improved weight-based alternative. PLoS One [Internet]. 2014;9(9):e108460. Available from: https://doi.org/10.1371/journal.pone.0108460.
21. Fields JB, Magee MK, Jones MT, Askow AT, Camic CL, Luedke J, et al. The accuracy of ten common resting metabolic rate prediction equations in men and women collegiate athletes. EJSS (Champaign) [Internet]. 2023;23(10):1973–82. Available from: https://doi.org/10.1080/17461391.2022.2130098.
22. Tinsley GM, Graybeal AJ, Moore ML. Resting metabolic rate in muscular physique athletes: validity of existing methods and development of new prediction equations. Appl Physiol Nutr Metab [Internet]. 2019;44(4):397–406. Available from: https://doi.org/10.1139/apnm-2018-0412.

Special Equations

5

Abstract

In clinical nutrition practice, energy estimation often centers on resting and total daily energy expenditure. However, alternative equations may be more appropriate when evaluating weight changes, energy availability for physical activity, or nutritional needs in critically ill individuals. This chapter explores the application of specialized formulas, including the ideal body weight (IBW) via the Devine formula, desired body weight, and the energy availability equation as complementary tools in nutritional assessment. Despite ongoing evaluation of their validity and reliability in the general population, these methods can enhance energy and macronutrient recommendations. Used in conjunction with standard equations, they provide a more comprehensive framework for clinicians seeking to optimize nutritional strategies across diverse patient populations.

Keywords

Lean body mass (LBM) · Weight loss · Energy availability (EA) · Low energy availability (LEA) · Ideal body weight (IBW)

S. Kitts, *Nutritional Assessment*,
https://doi.org/10.1007/978-3-032-22506-1_5

Learning Objectives
By the end of this chapter, students should be able to:

- Describe the purpose and application of alternative energy estimation equations, including ideal body weight (IBW), desired body weight, and the energy availability equation.
- Analyze the limitations, validity concerns, and contextual appropriateness of alternative equations compared to more rigorously validated predictive models.
- Evaluate how combining alternative equations with standard methods (e.g., BMI, REE/TDEE equations) enhances the comprehensiveness of nutritional assessment.
- Apply alternative formulas to case examples to estimate energy or macronutrient needs in diverse patient populations.

The use of alternative equations may need to be considered when practitioners are not looking to calculate resting or total daily energy estimates. The equations that will be discussed in this chapter will focus on other equations that help to evaluate weight changes, energy availability for activity, and assess weight for those with critical illnesses. Although these equations are still being evaluated for validity and reliability in general population, they can be a helpful tool for assessing the energy and macronutrient needs of an individual. More importantly, these special equations can be used in conjunction with the other equations to provide more information for nutritional assessment.

For this chapter, the same example individual and data block will be utilized.

Data Block (for the Chapter)

Gender	Female	Additional information and conversions
Age	42	
Height	5′6″	66 in/1.67 m/2.82 m^2/167.64 cm
Weight	180	81.82 kg

Gender	Female	Additional information and conversions
Physical activity level (PAL)	1.6	She has been trying to lose weight over the past 6 months. Physical activity is 5 days/week, 30–35 min of moderate intensity
% body fat	36%	Measured by calipers method

Ideal Body Weight (IBW) to the Devine Formula

Background The Metropolitan Life Insurance Company created height and weight tables for the sole purpose of life insurance underwriting. Published versions started in 1942, and the last published table was in 1983. At the time, the tables were used by the company to assess an individual's risk and set the premiums for life insurance [1]. The premise for these tables was that the "ideal" weight for individuals could be associated with the lowest mortality rate risk. The methodology or correlation that these tables used to rate policyholders were criticized as it oversimplified the relationship between body composition and body frame size. Additionally, the data that was used to build these tables included predominantly white, middle-class individuals and did not account for body composition. The charts have now been replaced with assessing BMI, and the insurance does not use weight as a determining factor for insurance policies.

The Devine formula was developed by BJ Devine in 1974 using the structure of the height-weight tables. The formula's original purpose was designed to standardize a method to estimate a patient's ideal weight to administer the proper drug dosage when the patient is obese [2]. Using total body weight to calculate drug dosages can lead to overdosing and potential toxicity, particularly for medications that do not distribute well into fat tissue.

The modern application of the Devine formula can be utilized with individuals participating in physical activity and athletic endeavors where it would be appropriate to set weight goals. For example, if an individual is setting a goal of losing weight as they have started a fitness plan or for an athlete that might be changing weight for their sport, like wrestling. When considering this formula, the practitioner should remember it is an estimate, and it is a starting point that should also factor in body composition and health outcomes.

Population The population for the Devine formula would be adults over five feet tall. The formula is not designed to be utilized with children, adolescents, and individuals that have large amounts of muscle mass or atypical body frames, anything varying from the medium frame size [2]. Additionally, in the clinical setting the formula still can be used to calculate dosages of medication for obese patients to avoid overdosage; however, more modern equations are preferred for clinical accuracy.

Validity and Limitations The validity for the Devine formula is limited and should be used for training or educational purposes to understand IBW calculations. The largest limitations of the Devine formula are the exclusion of body composition, muscle mass, bone density, and physical activity energy requirements.

Equation
Males: 50 kg + 2.3 kg per inch over 5 feet
Females: 45.5 kg + 2.3 kg per inch over 5 feet

Example:
45.5 kg + 2.3 kg per inch over 5 feet
45.5 kg + (2.3 kg × 6 inches)
45.5 kg + 13.8 kg = 59.3 kg
59.3 × 2.2 = 130.46 lbs (conversion back to pounds)

Desired Body Weight Formula

Background The American Council on Exercise (ACE) created a desired body weight (DBW) formula that utilizes an individual's current lean body mass and a desired body fat percentage. The

ACE organization promotes healthy living through educating, training, and certifying fitness professionals. The DBW formula can assist in helping individuals set realistic goals for weight loss or a target weight. This formula is a simple tool that should be considered as a starting point of discussion about current weight and how to safely plan weight loss goals.

Population The DBW formula can be used on adult populations that are overweight or obese and discuss appropriate weight loss based on a percentage of body weight. However, there are very clear populations in the DBW formula that should not be used with the following populations: muscular individuals and athletes, individuals with chronic health issues, and adolescents and teenagers. These populations will need other calculations that will address their specific needs and health concerns.

Validity and Limitations The DBW formula offers a practical method for estimating target weight, but it should be interpreted as a flexible guideline rather than a goal. Its accuracy can vary significantly between individuals due to unaccounted factors such as muscle mass, bone density, and genetic variability. As a result, modern assessment strategies increasingly favor body composition analysis to provide a more personalized and precise evaluation of weight-related health goals.

Ultimately, there are a couple of considerations for using the DBW formula for individuals to be successful. First, the DBW formula will assume that the individual will only lose fat mass and maintain lean mass as they lose weight. Muscle losses are detrimental during weight loss, therefore weight loss should be slow and monitored to preserve muscle. Second, mathematically the DBW formula provides a guideline or baseline, not a precise number for the targeted weight loss number. This number may vary and change when the percentage of body fat changes. ACE has moved away from using this formula alone due to the single use of inaccuracy and reliance on an individual's perfect body fat. Protocols for ACE professionals now utilize multiple health assessments to give individuals a more holistic approach to a health assessment. Assessments can include the DBW formula in conjunction with BMI and hip-to-waist ratios. Overall, the DBW formula offers an educational opportunity and a place to start conversations about proper weight loss changes.

Equation

Desired Body Weight (DBW)

DBW = LBW ÷ (1 − DBF%)

Step 1: 100% − Fat % = Lean body %

Step 2: Body weight × Lean body % = LBW

Step 3: 100% − Desired fat % = Desired lean %

Step 4: LBW ÷ Desired lean % = DBW

Example:

Step 1: 100% − 36% = 64% (LB%)

Step 2: 180 lbs × 0.64 = 115.2 (LBW)

Step 3: 100% − 31% = 69% (Desired Lean %)

Step 4: **115.2 LBW/69% (Desired Lean %) = 166.96 lbs**

Energy Availability Equation

Background The concept of energy availability (EA) has evolved from its initial concept in determining mammalian physiological energy needs to wide use in exercise science today. In broad nutrition terms, EA is described as the amount of dietary energy that remains after physical activity that will fulfill all other metabolic processes. Therefore, this formula can explain EA by determining the difference between the energy intake (EI) and the exercise energy expenditure (EEE) in relation to an individual's lean body mass (LBM) [3]. The importance of this equation can help to identify athletes that may be increasing exercise (outgoing calories), possibly have reduced energy intake (incoming calories), or have the possibility of these happening simultaneously. If these scenarios, singularly or together, are occurring, the individual could be at risk for hormonal, endocrinological, and metabolic dysregulations [4]. This will be discussed; however, there are two important parts to this equation: evolution of the equation and the required variables.

Evolution of the EA Equation The earliest investigations into EA focused on the physiological adaptations due to exercise and nutrition. The current concept of EA in the late twentieth century focused on the relationship between the variables of EA, EI, and EEE. From this research spawned the concept of the 30 kcal/kg/day threshold wherein females could have a critical cut-off or risk acceleration of menstrual disturbances [5]. The mechanism for this theory focuses on EA dropping below the 30 kcal/kg/day threshold of fat-free mass (FFM) disrupting hormones and menstrual cycles. As this concept also evolved, with the influence of individual physiological and activity variabilities, the threshold should be interpreted as an increased risk for disruption, not a strict cutoff. Modern research of the EA measurement examines the acute and chronic effects of low energy availability (LEA) on muscle protein synthesis and other metabolic/physiological pathways [4]. The chart below shows the evolution of the EA formula and important points of distinction (Table 5.1).

Table 5.1 Evolution of the EA formula

	Formula	Information
First algebraic definition	$EA = (EI - TEEE)/BW$ $EA = (EI{-}TEEE)/BW$ (Total energy expenditure)	First equation for humans and provided a quantifiable parameter
Second algebraic definition	$EA = (EI - TEEE)/LBM$	The equation was refined to account for the "energy balance" concept by adjusting lean body mass (LBM) instead of body weight
Third algebraic definition	$EA = (EI - EEE)/LBM$ $EA = (EI - EEE)/LBM$	EEE is calculated by subtracting non-exercise energy expenditure

Required Variables The EA equation has three variables that are required to find the individual's EA. Each of these variables has been previously highlighted in the background information; however, not explained where to find them or their importance.

1. Energy Intake (EI)—for this variable, the individuals will need to provide their total energy calories per day. This could be self-reported from the individual that tracks calories or calculated from an energy expenditure estimate.
2. Exercise Energy Expenditure (EEE)—this variable will require a measurement either by a direct method (metabolic measurement) or indirect method (heart rate monitors, pedometers, or self-report tools). Some activities or sports might need to be calculated based on metabolic equivalents (METs). The MET values for specific sports can also be found from sources like the Compendium of Physical Activities.
3. Fat-Free Mass (FFM)—the variable will be calculated by subtracting the individual's fat mass from their body weight to obtain the FFM in kilograms. This weight would include muscle, bones, organs, and water in the body.

The EA equation offers a valuable framework for assessing nutritional adequacy in relation to physical activity by utilizing the three variables. EI is accessible but often imprecise due to self-reporting errors; EEE can be tailored to specific activities but varies in accuracy depending on the measurement method; and FFM provides essential context for individual energy needs but requires reliable body composition assessment. Understanding these nuances is critical for interpreting EA values and identifying at-risk individuals.

Population The importance of this equation furthered the investigation of insufficient EA and the effects of low energy availability (LEA) on a broader issue of relative energy deficiency in sport (RED-S). When athletes do not consume enough total energy to support basic metabolic needs and physical activity for sport, deficiencies develop; the athlete could be at a higher risk of injury and could suffer from poor performances [5]. RED-S was previously known as the "Female Athlete Triad," which eliminated the possibility that males could also suffer from LEA. This was an important advancement in the assessment of all athletes to focus on the physiology and health functions that are associated with athletic performance.

However, the Female Athlete Triad is still an important consideration in the LEA for female athletes. Historically, the Triad was defined by the American College of Sports Medicine (ACSM) in 1992 as disordered eating pattern, amenorrhea (loss of menstrual cycle for three or more months), and osteoporotic changes [6]. Since then, research has recognized that these three interrelated components should be viewed on a continuum or spectrum. This would allow for individual variances between eumenorrhea (normal menstruation) and amenorrhea, optimal bone health and osteoporosis, and optimal EA and LEA with or without the presence of an eating disorder (ED) [6]. This approach allows for a more accurate representation of where the individual may present components along the spectrum.

Validity and Limitations The EA equation validity presents some limitations; however, the practicality to relay the negative impact of a calorie deficiency on athlete's health and performance is important. The validity can be seen in the evidence from the vast research that has utilized the formula. The evolution of the formula has found the link between LEA below the 30 kcal/kg of fat-free mass per day and altering hormonal and metabolic issues in female athletes. Additionally, the EA equation has increased the communication of EA in males and females by raising the awareness of under fueling and performance consequences [7]. The establishing of healthy values (45 kcal/kg/day threshold of FFM) and the problematic health consideration (below 30 kcal/kg/day threshold of FFM) create a logical soundness needed to describe the relationship.

Still, the limitations for the EA equation will focus on the lack of accuracy of the variables. The first limitation comes from the lack of a uniform interpretation of total exercise expenditure [7].

As discussed earlier in this text, the accuracy of calculating EEE varies widely due to the activity or sport being estimated, self-reporting calories from trackers, or established calculated energy estimation for general activities. Errors that are reported are from either under- or overreporting of calories expended, which do not account for intensity levels sometimes. Next, energy consumption of calories within the diet is also known to be self-reported, which can result in underreporting. Interestingly, the use of self-reported food records has shown up to 60% of errors from the underreporting of total calories [7]. This can be a significant hurdle to overcome with a formula that requires this main variable. Finally, there is a lack of a universal threshold of concern or a cut-off value [7]. Within this limitation, consider individual variability, gender differences, and the inability to consider an adaptable vs. problematic LEA for an athlete. These three considerations speak to the variations between athletes; for example, one athlete may be experiencing a small dip in calories without any negative LEA effects. Whereas another athlete may experience the manifestation of some health consequences from a small dip in calories. Therefore, the EA formula cannot predict a problematic calorie deficit in a single snapshot.

Equation

Athletes' kg – %BF = LBM

Energy intake – training calories = Residual energy

Residual energy/LBM = Energy availability

Compare to critical cutoff – is it appropriate for athlete

It should be noted that there will be two new information points required for this formula.

- (Energy intake according to Chap. 4 assessment of total estimated energy = 2401 kcal)
- (Training calories for 35 min of moderate training on elliptical or treadmill = 350 kcal)
- Also, the %BF will be determined by finding the FFM. ($81.82 \times 0.36 = 29.47$)

Example –
81.82 – 29.47 = 52.39 LBM
2401 – 350 = 2051 Residual energy
2051/52.39 = 39.15 Energy availability (Appropriate EA)

Chapter Summary

The use of these alternative equations may lack scientific rigor when compared to the equations in Chap. 4. However, these equations can play a practical and useful purpose in guiding clinicians and individuals to gather all related data for the nutritional assessment. By scientific definition, a valid equation should be logically sound and mathematically consistent; it will provide an accurate representation of relationships. Although the limitations for each of these equations are noted, the usefulness of providing sufficient accuracy or approximation for the distinct purpose of an assessment. The special formulas could be used in conjunction with BMI and estimating energy equations to give a greater picture to the individual. Therefore, the use of IBW or Devine Formula, desired body weight formula from ACE, and the energy availability formula may lack theoretical validity but provide a practical means to illustrate underlying principles. The contextual validity of these simplified formulas will provide valuable insights and predictions to be used for pedagogical reasons. Ultimately, the use of multiple approaches will ensure a more holistic review.

Chapter Review Questions

1. What are the major limitations of these specialized formulas, and how do concerns about validity and reliability affect their use in general populations?
2. In what ways can alternative equations complement standard energy estimation methods to create a more holistic nutritional assessment?

3. How can the Devine IBW formula or Desired Body Weight formula assist clinicians in evaluating weight changes or setting nutrition-related goals?
4. Why is practitioner familiarity with multiple equations important, and how does combining several data points (e.g., BMI, body composition, activity level) improve the accuracy of nutrition recommendations?

References

1. Weigley ES. Average? Ideal? Desirable? A brief overview of height-weight tables in the United States. J Am Diet Assoc [Internet]. 1984;84(4):417–23. Available from: https://doi.org/10.1016/s0002-8223(21)08170-0.
2. Pai MP, Paloucek FP. The origin of the "ideal" body weight equations. Ann Pharmacother [Internet]. 2000;34(9):1066–9. Available from: https://doi.org/10.1345/aph.19381.
3. Loucks AB. Exercise training in the normal female: effects of low energy availability on reproductive function. In: Endocrinology of physical activity and sport. Cham: Springer International Publishing; 2020. p. 171–91.
4. Areta JL, Taylor HL, Koehler K. Low energy availability: history, definition and evidence of its endocrine, metabolic and physiological effects in prospective studies in females and males. Eur J Appl Physiol [Internet]. 2021;121(1):1–21. Available from: https://doi.org/10.1007/s00421-020-04516-0.
5. Mountjoy M, Sundgot-Borgen J, Burke L, Carter S, Constantini N, Lebrun C, et al. The IOC consensus statement: beyond the female athlete triad–relative energy deficiency in sport (RED-S). Br J Sports Med [Internet]. 2014;48(7):491–7. Available from: https://doi.org/10.1136/bjsports-2014-093502.
6. Kelly AW, Hecht S. The female athlete triad. Ann Jt [Internet]. 2022 [cited 2025 Oct 26];7(0):6. Available from: https://aoj.amegroups.org/article/view/6345/html
7. Jeukendrup AE, Areta JL, Van Genechten L, Langan-Evans C, Pedlar CR, Rodas G, et al. Does relative energy deficiency in sport (REDs) syndrome exist? Sports Med [Internet]. 2024;54(11):2793–816. Available from: https://doi.org/10.1007/s40279-024-02108-y.

Nutrient Requirements

6

Abstract

This chapter examines the role of macronutrients in meeting nutrient requirements and maintaining overall health. Current dietary recommendations provide general population guidelines for the distribution of carbohydrates, proteins, and fats, highlighting their essential functions in energy provision, growth, and repair. The assessment of macronutrient intake emphasizes both quality and quantity, recognizing that nutrient-dense sources support health while excesses of refined or imbalanced intake may increase disease risk. While standardized ratios such as the acceptable macronutrient distribution ranges (AMDR) offer a framework for population-level guidance, individual differences that include activity level and health status necessitate personalized approaches. This chapter underscores the importance of balancing current recommendations with individualized macronutrient ratios to optimize dietary strategies, ensuring both adequacy and diet sustainability.

Keywords

Macronutrients · Nutrient recommendations · Excessive consumption · Health outcomes · Nitrogen balance · Weight management · Distribution ranges

S. Kitts, *Nutritional Assessment*,
https://doi.org/10.1007/978-3-032-22506-1_6

Learning Objectives

By the end of this chapter students should be able to:

- Describe the essential functions of carbohydrates, proteins, and fats in supporting energy needs, growth, repair, and overall health.
- Explain the purpose and application of the acceptable macronutrient distribution ranges (AMDR) and how they guide population-level dietary recommendations.
- Evaluate the impact of nutrient quality versus quantity, including how nutrient-dense versus refined sources affect health outcomes and disease risk.
- Apply estimated energy requirements and dietary guidelines to calculate individualized macronutrient needs in grams and percentages.
- Assess the role of nutrition education, reliable information sources, and public health guidelines in shaping healthy eating patterns and managing misinformation.

The initial steps of a health history and estimated energy requirements have been assessed as the next step of nutrient requirements becomes the focus. There are many established sources for educating individuals on their nutrient requirements and how to manage the nutrients in their diet. However, lack of dietary education and the perpetuation of social media trends or misinformation can greatly hinder a healthy diet. Breaking down the basics of macro- and micronutrients can empower individuals to make informed choices and improve decision-making to establish healthy eating patterns. Another important piece to convey to individuals is where to find information from reliable sources. Empowering individuals with this information will shape healthy eating habits.

The intent of this chapter is not to go in depth on each macronutrient, but rather to offer the current dietary guidelines utilized in the healthcare field and how the information can be applied on an individual basis. Macronutrient information will utilize the current guidelines from the United States Department of Agriculture (USDA) has a long history of monitoring and researching nutrition information for the American population. In fact, since 1894 the USDA updates the dietary guidelines every five years to reflect current research and health trends. Dietary recommendations will continue to evolve as eating patterns change; however, the focus of eliminating deficiencies and improving health outcomes remains.

Current Nutrient Recommendations

The guidelines use scientific proof to advise on healthy diets for everyone in the United States, from healthy people to those who have or are at risk for diet-related diseases [1]. The 2020–2025 guidelines highlight four key guidelines and four additional recommendations that should be considered for the American population. The four overarching guidelines focus on healthy diet through all life stages, incorporating and customizing diet to fit personal preferences (culturally and budgetarily), focusing on nutrient density without exceeding total calorie limits, and limiting added sugars, saturated fats, sodium, and alcoholic beverages. These guidelines are reasonable for dietary changes or adjustments for individuals to make. Education for individuals will be essential as incorporating nutrient-dense without exceeding total calorie consumption will need to be practiced. Understanding the terms alone can cause confusion about how to determine the total calorie limit. The use of the estimated energy equations can help visualize where calories come from the daily diet.

The USDA also has four key recommendations that support the guidelines based on the scientific quantitative evidence they have collected. These four recommendations give individuals specific numerical goals to consider (Table 6.1).

The 2020–2025 guidelines continued earlier guidance in the areas noted; however, this was the first time that the USDA incorporated stage of life recommendations and the inclusion of personal or cultural aspects to the guidelines. Including recommendations like these show the adaptability of the guidelines to a larger population, incorporating dietary changes to improve health outcomes.

Table 6.1 USDA current recommendations for Americans Dietaryguidelines.gov [1]

Additive sugars should be limited to less than 10% of calories per day for ages 2 and older, with a further designation of avoiding additive sugars for infants and toddlers
For individuals aged 2 and older, saturated fats should be less than 10% of total calories consumed per day
Sodium intake should be less than 2300 mg per day
Limiting or moderation of alcoholic drinks per day

Other considerations that are discussed in this current guideline cycle include varying protein sources, maintaining a healthy weight, and incorporating more plant-based items into the diet plan. These are helpful additions that can provide essential vitamins, minerals, and other health-promoting components without the addition of unwanted sugar, saturated fats, and sodium. Education about how an individual plans their diet can be done here explaining the differences between processed versus ultra-processed foods. For example, incorporating more plant-based foods will reduce overall processing of food sources, thereby eliminating extra calories and unwanted sugar, saturated fats, and sodium.

Macronutrient Assessment

Macronutrient assessment is used in a nutrition assessment to help determine the balance of carbohydrates, proteins, and fats in an individual's diet. This process ensures that they meet their energy and health needs and determine whether the nutrients align with the dietary guidelines. An assessment will require calculating an individual's daily caloric needs and then determining an optimal distribution of the macronutrients. Once the distribution is found, the macronutrient need can be expressed as grams or a percentage of total calories for the individual to see full picture. It is important for individuals that have specific dietary goals such as weight management, muscle growth, or managing medial conditions like diabetes to have this breakdown information for dietary planning.

This information can then be incorporated into online macronutrient calculators or food/calorie tracking apps to help individual monitor day-to-day intakes. The calculated assessment or online/app estimates should be used as a starting point as individual's results and feedback may warrant adjustments in the distributions. Ultimately, the quantity and quality of macronutrients will be determined by the individual's current diet and where changes can be made.

Diving deeper into the macronutrient assessment, each plays a vital role in bodily functions to maintain an optimal balance for overall health. This becomes an important education element for individuals to understand that imbalances, deficiencies, and overages can affect the balance of macronutrients, which can directly affect health. Therefore, explaining each macronutrient's function in the body will be important for individuals to see their essential worth and variations can impact healthy functions.

Carbohydrates are the body's primary source of energy and preferred source of energy within the cells. The simplest carbohydrates are glucose, which is energy that can be used immediately as it travels through the blood system. The brain, central nervous system, and muscles utilize glucose or stored form glycogen in muscles or liver for energy at the cellular level. The energy value or currency of carbohydrates is 4 calories of energy per gram (4 kcal/g). The most complex carbohydrate fiber is an indigestible component that has direct correlation to healthy digestion, bowel function, and overall health outcomes.

Excess carbohydrates and diets that supply chronic overconsumption can lead to weight gain, obesity, and an increased risk of type 2 diabetes [2]. The process of storing glycogen will reach a limit or full capacity, and the excess will be converted to fat in the liver and stored in the body. Specifically, the body will convert the glucose into fatty acids and glycerol which are further converted to triglycerides in the fat cells.

Finding the balance of carbohydrates and focusing on the type of carbohydrates will be essential to increase health outcomes. The worth of a carbohydrate can be explained by increasing the complexity of the source (increasing fiber) and also increasing the worth of overall health. Starch and fiber carbohydrate sources have direct health outcomes in the promotion of satiety or fullness, reducing cholesterol levels, gut health, and immune function [3].

Proteins are considered the primary building blocks of body cells. The largest function of protein is to provide a supply of amino acids to provide mechanical and structural purposes that support the health of the body [3]. For example, amino acids are utilized to build, repair, and maintain tissues in the body such as muscle, skin, and organ tissues. The energy value or currency of proteins is also 4 calories of energy per gram (4 kcal/g) and contains nitrogen, which the other two macronutrients do not. The addition of nitrogen is the essential piece of amino acids being the fundamental building blocks. Therefore, protein has critical roles in creating enzymes, forming hormones and antibodies, regulating chemical reactions, and supporting immune function.

Excess protein through dietary consumption is complex because the body does not store protein efficiently and poses a larger metabolic risk to the kidneys and liver [2]. The body will process excess protein through four avenues:

1. Deamination—a metabolic process of removing an amino acid group.
2. Energy production—through gluconeogenesis in the liver will convert excessive amino acids into glucose or fat. This is not a direct pathway for energy and considered to be a slower process or essential in times where the body is under stress, low blood sugar, or a fasting state.
3. Fat storage—because the body does not have a dedicated or specialized storage cell to store excess protein, it will need to be converted to a fatty acid for ultimate storage as triglycerides in adipose tissues. This type of fatty acid synthesis from amino acids happens when there is an excess and accompanies high insulin levels [4]. This is not an ideal mechanism for energy and should be used as a last resort reserve.
4. Waste removal—the removed amino acid group is converted to ammonia and then urea, which can be excreted from the body via kidneys. Excretion of waste from the metabolism of protein will increase the strain on the kidney and could lead to dehydration.

It should be noted that there is much debate about how much protein can be taken during one meal or sitting. Research in protein ingestion post-exercise in trained individuals may not have a limit, as these individuals have a need for protein due to the metabolic stress of exercise [5]. The overarching advice is that everyone, from sedentary to active individuals, needs sufficient dietary protein. To achieve this, a distribution and variety of protein sources throughout the day are evident, not focusing on a single meal amount. Lastly, physical activity levels will be the determining factor in overall consumption and usage of amino acids.

Nitrogen balance is a way to describe protein metabolism and determine protein requirements. The body tries to achieve a nitrogen balance by maintaining the amount of protein (+ nitrogen) consumed equaling the amount of protein (– nitrogen) that will be excreted. When nitrogen exceeds nitrogen loss, this is considered a positive (anabolic) state where the body is building or repairing bodily tissues, in growth periods, healing injuries, or undergoing strenuous physical activity. When the flip of this scenario happens, nitrogen loss is greater than caloric intake, this is a negative state where the body is breaking down (catabolic) tissues due to malnutrition, starvation, illness, or injury from overtraining or excessive physical activity.

Fats are also termed lipids or dietary fats, which have the most calorie-dense energy when compared to the other two macronutrients. The energy value or currency of lipids is 9 calories of energy per gram (9 kcal/g) and will serve as the main form of stored energy in the body. Lipids serve as essential pieces of several physiological pathways such as production of sex hormones, body temperature regulation, cell structure, and transportation and absorption of fat-soluble vitamins A, D, E, and K [2]. There are several different forms of dietary fats that should be considered:

1. Triglycerides—composed of a glycerol backbone and has three fatty acids attached to it. They make up sources such as fats and oils.
2. Phospholipids—a major component of cell membranes as they consist of a hydrophilic head and a hydrophobic tail, thereby

creating and bilayer structure. These are crucial for brain and nerve health and can be found in egg yolks, soy, and seeds.
3. Sterols (cholesterol)—can be found in either animal cell membranes or plants. These lipids help to maintain cell membranes and are the precursors for some hormones. They can be found in meats, nuts, seeds, and margarine.
4. Fatty acids—are considered the building blocks of fat. Once they are broken down from food, they can be used as an energy source and can form cell membranes. Found in butter, milk, beef, and oils.

Diets that are high in fat in the body will readily store in the body's fat cells. Long-term excessive intakes of a high-fat diet can manifest fat accumulation throughout the body and an increased risk of metabolic diseases. Diseases associated with increased risk of weight gain, obesity, cardiovascular disease, type 2 diabetes, and some cancers [6]. Additionally, diets that have higher levels of saturated fats are linked to higher cholesterol levels and higher values of low-density lipoproteins (LDL) or bad cholesterol.

Although there are several negative associations with fat and health, the types of fats are most important as they do play a role in overall health. Replacing the saturated fats could be done with unsaturated fats as they are considered more heart protective. Additionally, fats such as omega-3s and docosahexaenoic acid (DHA), a component of omega-3s, are necessary for brain health, cognitive function, and hormone production.

The macronutrient assessment requires the practitioners to know the function and the possible impacts if the diet provides excess or deficient amounts of carbohydrates, protein, and fats. It is finding the right combination or balance of the macronutrients for individuals to maintain essential overall health goals. When one macronutrient is the focus or overfocus of an individual's diet (protein), there will be a natural decrease in another (carbohydrate), which can have impacts on chronic disease risk and micronutrient levels.

The education of the macronutrient balance is the sticking point; incorporating foods that share macronutrients is an excellent way to increase the complexity of the foods an individual is eating. For example, for individuals that want complex fiber-based carbohydrates that also have protein, they can incorporate beans/lentils, quinoa, nuts, and oatmeal. This is an important concept to consider; most mainstream information will push direct sources of protein (animal-based) which will also have a higher fat content and decrease the needed complex carbohydrates. Plant-based proteins are considered incomplete due to lacking one or more of the nine essential amino acids; however, eating diverse sources of incomplete proteins is beneficial for the fiber. Pairing complex carbohydrates with a variety of complete and incomplete protein throughout the day is a goal for individuals to consider. Concepts like this will help to shape the individual's macronutrient assessment for further education on how to properly distribute the nutrients throughout the diet.

Distribution of Macronutrients

Macronutrient distribution is the requirement of portions of carbohydrates, proteins, and fats needed in an individual's total daily energy intake. This is very dependent on many factors that include age, activity levels, and medical conditions, which in turn become variables for determining the distribution. Understanding which variables need to be accounted for can help to reduce overeating, provide calories for physical activity, and support changes in weight. Therefore, the following reasons show the importance of distributing macronutrients based on individual considerations.

1. Weight management—an appropriate distribution of macronutrients can help to regulate weight gains, losses, or maintenance by reducing cravings, maintaining satiety or fullness after eating, and sustained energy.
2. Energy and metabolism—consumption of calories from a variety of sources can maintain sustained energy levels and support activity. In addition, those individuals that are maintaining or increasing muscle mass may need to adjust macronutrients to support goals.

3. Health changes—in times when there is an illness or injury, changes may be needed to support tissue repair or the immune system.
4. Individual specific goals—individuals that have a goal of weight gains or losses will require different distributions and ratios. For example, weight loss versus weight gain through increasing muscle mass will have to consider total calories and distribution.

Using the variables, calculation of how many grams of each macronutrient is needed for an individual will help create the distribution. There can also be an estimate of the proportions required and how they can be ingested differently daily. The general daily percentages of each macronutrient include carbohydrates at 45–65% of total daily calories, protein at 10–35% of total daily calories, and fats at 20–35% of total daily calories [7]. These percentages are recommended under the standards of the Dietary Guidelines for Americans as part of the 2025–2030 current reporting cycle.

This final considerations for macronutrient distribution are individual needs and food quality. As previously discussed, individual needs will be determined during the assessment and will be based on their overall health, activity levels, genetics, and goals. The next section of macronutrient ratios will address this more as personalization can be tackled there. Food quality has not been discussed in the distribution of macronutrients. However, the concept of increasing nutrient density or worth of foods to supply necessary vitamins, minerals, and total calories has been found. Utilizing diets that are more plant-based and less processed foods can be important in considering the total calories and quality of the macronutrients.

Macronutrient Ratios

The macronutrient ratios are for the population to consider dietary plans to be structured. The amounts of each macronutrient that should be eaten to maintain a healthy weight or health outcomes. There is no ideal for every person or population. Having a range of guidance provides an effective way to calculate the grams, which helps put the food intake of individuals into perspective and able to determine where adjustments need to be made if necessary.

There are many different ratios in the general population; an example may be shown as 45:30:25 (carbohydrate, protein, fat). Additionally, different ratios that will accommodate athletes, individuals with medical conditions, and ethnic backgrounds, which include differences in genetics and diverse cultural lifestyles, can be used for macronutrient ratios. The following chart summarizes common macronutrient ratios utilized in various areas of health care, physical fitness, and dietary guidelines (Table 6.2):

Table 6.2 Recommended macronutrient distributions for specified populations

Acceptable Macronutrient Distribution Range (AMDR) [8]	Wider ranges to accommodate population and varying needs	Carbohydrates: 45–65% Protein: 10–35% Fats: 20–35%
Weight Loss Distribution Range [9]	Suggestion for caloric reduction and higher protein to minimize muscle loss	Carbohydrates: 40–50% Proteins: 30% Fats: 20–30%
Muscle gain/ Body Building [10]	Specific ratios based on individual goals and training phase	Carbohydrates: 45–60% Proteins: 25–30% Fats: 15–25%
Endurance athletes [11]	Suggested to increase carbohydrates to replenish glycogen stores	Carbohydrates: 55–65% Protein: 20–30% Fat: 20–30%
Injured or post-surgical [12]	Suggested to increase omega-3 fatty acids to enhance anabolism (growth & repair)	Carbohydrates: 45–65% Protein 15–25% Fats: 10–35%
Illness or chronic disease state [13]	Must be adjusted based on specific conditions, increasing plant-based and focus on healthy fats	Carbohydrates: 45–65% Protein: 10–35% Fats: 20–35% Eliminating or minimizing saturated fats and trans-fats

These recommendations are general guidelines and will require a personalized distribution configuration and monitoring when changes are needed. Considerations of established meals or dietary patterns will help the individual make changes in an appropriate way. Therefore, manipulating the ratios effectively for individuals will require practice and incorporating personal goals into the plan. The steps to strategically plan the distribution of the macronutrients should include:

1. Collection of health history, anthropometrics, and disease assessment
   - This information will help providers to understand specific needs of individuals.
   - Also, provide information on objective goals: weight loss, decreasing risk of disease, weight gain, or weight maintenance.
2. Calculate total daily calories needed
   - Use the appropriate estimated energy equation to set a daily calorie target.
3. Choose a target ratio
   - Start with a macronutrient ratio that addresses individual's goals and specific activity needs.
4. Calculate the grams needed for each macronutrient per day
   - Using the determined percentages, convert into daily grams by using the energy yield for each macronutrient.
   - Carbohydrate 4 cal/g, Protein 4 cal/g, and Fat 9 cal/g
5. Track and monitor the individual's progress
   - Tracking can be achieved through food journals, online sources, and apps.
   - Monitoring the individual's objective goals, such as weight changes and measurements, and subjective information, feelings, or feedback.
6. Adjust total calories and ratios gradually
   - Subjective information on how they are feeling daily, after exercise, and any fatigue can be important information on energy levels.

- Small adjustments in calories or specific macronutrients can affect total daily energy or availability of nutrients to the body.

7. Emphasize the overall quality of the diet
   - Focusing on nutrient dense and wide variety of food sources is most important.
   - Quality and quantity of macro- and micronutrients will be beneficial.

This strategic plan is less about rigid formulas and more about tailoring macronutrient ratios to the individual. Starting by understanding a person's health history and goals, then setting calorie targets that reflect daily energy needs. From there, macronutrient ratios are chosen to match activity demands, whether that means higher carbohydrates for endurance athletes or protein strength gains. Macronutrient ratios can be tailored to individuals who are injured, ill, or recovering too. Distinction of the individual's health state and activity level is a needed component. Then these ratios are translated into grams per day, making them actionable for diet planning. Progress is tracked not only through numbers like weight or measurements but also through how the individual feels by evaluating energy levels, recovery, and fatigue in all guide adjustments. Small tweaks in calories or macronutrient distribution can make a big difference, and the emphasis always comes back to diet quality: nutrient-dense foods, variety, and balance. In practice, this approach ensures that nutrition strategies are flexible, personalized, and sustainable rather than "one size fits all" recommendations.

Individual Ratios Versus General Population

The AMDR was developed to provide greater population guidance on macronutrient ranges associated with appropriate intake and decreasing risk for disease. General population information is valuable for public health, policy, and resources to reach everyone. This is where the information can be disseminated to the greatest extent possible; however, it doesn't address the individual's specific needs. The two are symbiotic in the sense that the knowledge that is shared by the general population can be adapted by individuals benefiting from the knowledge while contributing to greater population. This is important as the adjustments can be made at each level to form future health strategies. Ultimately, the general ratios are seen as the foundation; personalizing the ratios will help individuals plan their diet and nutrition from the ground up.

Chapter Summary

This chapter explores the nutrient requirements and the role of macronutrients in health and performance. Current dietary recommendations provide general guidance for energy and nutrient intake, emphasizing balanced proportions of carbohydrates, proteins, and fats to support physiological functions. The quality of macronutrient intake is as important as the quantity. Nutrient-dense sources such as whole grains, lean proteins, and unsaturated fats promote health, while excesses of simple carbohydrates, saturated and trans fats, or protein beyond needs can contribute to disease risk. Assessing macronutrient intake therefore requires attention to both adequacy and moderation.

Distribution of macronutrients is typically guided by established ranges, such as the Acceptable Macronutrient Distribution Ranges (AMDR), which recommend 45–65% of calories from carbohydrates, 10–35% from protein, and 20–35% from fat. These ratios provide a framework for population-level health, but individual needs often differ. Athletes, individuals with chronic conditions, or those with specific body composition goals may require tailored macronutrient ratios that deviate from general recommendations.

Ultimately, nutrition planning balances general population guidelines with individualized approaches. While standardized ratios offer a useful starting point, effective dietary strategies must account for personal health history, activity level, and metabolic differences. This chapter underscores the importance of both evidence-based recommendations and personalized adjustments to achieve optimal health outcomes.

Chapter Review Questions

1. What are the primary functions of each macronutrient, and why are both quality and quantity important when assessing macronutrient intake?
2. How do the Acceptable Macronutrient Distribution Ranges (AMDR) support population-level dietary guidance, and what limitations arise when applying them to individuals?
3. After estimating an individual's daily caloric needs, how would you determine an appropriate macronutrient distribution, and how can this be expressed in both grams and percentages?
4. Which individual variables (e.g., age, activity level, medical conditions) most strongly influence macronutrient requirements, and how do these variables guide personalized dietary planning?
5. In what ways do population-level dietary guidelines and individualized nutrition strategies complement one another, and why are both necessary for effective health promotion?

References

1. U.S. Department of Agriculture and U.S. Department of Health and Human Services. Dietary Guidelines for Americans, 2020–2025. 9th ed. Dietary Guidelines for Americans (.gov); 2020.
2. Espinosa-Salas S, Gonzalez-Arias M. Nutrition: macronutrient intake, imbalances, and interventions. In: StatPearls. Treasure Island: StatPearls Publishing; 2025.
3. Cena H, Calder PC. Defining a healthy diet: evidence for the role of contemporary dietary patterns in health and disease. Nutrients [Internet]. 2020;12(2):334. Available from: https://doi.org/10.3390/nu12020334.
4. Nakrani MN, Wineland RH, Anjum F. Physiology, glucose metabolism. In: StatPearls. Treasure Island: StatPearls Publishing; 2025.

5. Witard OC, Mettler S. The anabolic response to protein ingestion during recovery from exercise has no upper limit in magnitude and duration in vivo in humans: a commentary. Int J Sport Nutr Exerc Metab [Internet]. 2024;34(5):322–4. Available from: https://doi.org/10.1123/ijsnem.2024-0041.
6. Wali JA, Jarzebska N, Raubenheimer D, Simpson SJ, Rodionov RN, O'Sullivan JF. Cardio-metabolic effects of high-fat diets and their underlying mechanisms-a narrative review. Nutrients [Internet]. 2020;12(5):1505. Available from: https://doi.org/10.3390/nu12051505.
7. Hhs U. Scientific Report of the 2025 Dietary guidelines advisory committee, Part E, Chapter 1.
8. National Academies of Sciences, Engineering, Medicine, Health, Medicine Division, Food, Nutrition Board. Description of the acceptable macronutrient distribution range. Washington, DC: National Academies Press; 2024.
9. Bellissimo N, Akhavan T. Effect of macronutrient composition on short-term food intake and weight loss. Adv Nutr [Internet]. 2015;6(3):302S–8S. Available from: https://doi.org/10.3945/an.114.006957.
10. Lambert CP, Frank LL, Evans WJ. Macronutrient considerations for the sport of bodybuilding. Sports Med [Internet]. 2004;34(5):317–27. Available from: https://doi.org/10.2165/00007256-200434050-00004.
11. Liu S, Hueglin S, Scaramella J, Vitale K. Performance-based nutrition for endurance training. In: Endurance sports medicine. Cham: Springer International Publishing; 2023. p. 387–410.
12. Papadopoulou SK. Rehabilitation nutrition for injury recovery of athletes: the role of macronutrient intake. Nutrients [Internet]. 2020;12(8):2449. Available from: https://doi.org/10.3390/nu12082449.
13. de Souza RJ, Swain JF, Appel LJ, Sacks FM. Alternatives for macronutrient intake and chronic disease: a comparison of the OmniHeart diets with popular diets and with dietary recommendations. Am J Clin Nutr [Internet]. 2008;88(1):1–11. Available from: https://doi.org/10.1093/ajcn/88.1.1.

Nutrition-Focused Recommendations

7

Abstract

This chapter explores the multidimensional process of developing nutrition-focused recommendations, emphasizing the integration of recommended guidelines, personal context, and behavioral psychology. Building upon nutritional assessments, the framework highlights four critical areas: health status and guidelines, personal preferences and lifestyle, foundational nutrition education, and behavioral and psychological aspects. These four areas will collectively shape individualized dietary strategies. Special attention is given to the psychological and behavioral factors influencing food choices, including environment, genetics, and culture, as well as the role of education in reinforcing sustainable change. Practical strategies such as portion control, nutrient-dense food selection, healthy swaps, and attention to hunger and satiety cues are tools for long-term success. By combining patient-centered approaches with multi-level interventions, this chapter underscores the importance of personalized, scalable recommendations that empower individuals to achieve improved health outcomes and reduce the risk of chronic disease.

Keywords

Nutritional education · Body composition · Physical activity Lifestyle considerations · Personal preference · Nutritional swaps · Nutrient-dense foods

S. Kitts, *Nutritional Assessment*,
https://doi.org/10.1007/978-3-032-22506-1_7

Learning Objectives:
By the end of this chapter students should be able to:

- Explain the four key areas of nutrition-focused recommendations: health status and guidelines, personal preferences and lifestyle, foundational nutrition education, and behavioral/psychological aspects.
- Evaluate the role of education in reinforcing behavioral change and promoting long-term sustainability of dietary interventions.
- Assess the potential impact of nutrition-focused recommendations on long-term health outcomes, including weight management and chronic disease prevention.
- Apply practical behavioral strategies, including portion control, nutrient-dense food selection, and hunger/satiety awareness, to individual educational scenarios.

The essential pieces of nutritional assessment have been assembled, and the individual puzzle is beginning to take shape. Nutrition-focused recommendation is the next step in creating a plan to identify and support individual goals. Recommendations for macronutrient intake require a personalized approach, a holistic review of an individual's lifestyle, and alignment with current evidence-based nutritional guidelines. Health providers can draw on four key areas to assess and tailor recommendations: health status and guidelines, personal preferences and lifestyle, foundational nutrition education, and behavioral and psychological aspects. Together, these areas create a multidimensional, personalized framework for education and the implementation of dietary changes, ensuring recommendations are both practical and sustainable.

Health Status and Guidelines

As previously discussed, a good health history will assess an individual's overall health status. However, reviewing their history and understanding their personal health objectives would be principal focus. Therefore, the first step would be to assess any medical conditions, existing or past, that should be accounted for or in need of management. For example, making nutritional recommendations for diabetes versus Crohn's disease is quite different and could require specific dietary modifications or considerations. Individuals with chronic disease can differ in the metabolic and physiological impacts and therefore would require a tailored dietary suggestion. This would not be a diet prescription, as only Registered Dietitians are qualified to make these recommendations; however, it would be a guideline of nutrient needs that should be considered to either reduce the risks or enhance the health outcomes. The following Table 7.1 shows the variances in diets based on health status [1, 2]:

Everyone will have to navigate these suggestions with the help of health professionals to find the nutritional plan that addresses specific needs and avoid complications. Every chronic condition

Table 7.1 Suggested nutrient needs by health status

Population	Dietary suggestions
General nutritional recommendations—healthy populations	Increase intake of fruits, vegetables, fiber, and lean proteins Limit saturated fats, added sugars, and alcohol Reduce sodium and processed foods
Cardiovascular disease	Reduce sodium Limit saturated fats, trans fats, and cholesterol Increase fiber, healthy oils, and potassium
Diabetes (type I)	Increase plant-based sources and whole grains Incorporate lean proteins and healthy fats Select low-fat dairy sources Avoid sugary drinks and processed foods
Diabetes (type II)	Increase plant-based sources and whole grains Limit added sugars and sugary drinks
Cancer	Increase fruits and vegetables for antioxidants Increase fiber Decrease processed foods and red meats
Irritable bowel syndrome	Increase soluble fiber Avoid insoluble fiber Focus on low-fat and less processed foods

comes with different presentations, focusing on the individuals' specific diagnosis and status of disease, and any coexisting conditions will help the overall outcome.

The next area to consider in the individual's health status is life cycle. Nutrition evolves throughout our life; there are times when total calories are very high to support growth patterns and then times when absorption or use of calories slows down. It can be challenging to navigate these changes; therefore, it is important to understand what the body requires and make good choices so that optimal health can be maintained. First, the nutritional requirement will vary by age, gender, and activity level. Second, at the core of the life cycle, nutritional requirements will focus on the differing needs of total calories, protein need, calcium, iron, vitamin D, and B complex [3]. These essential requirements of the diet in addition to hydration levels will support overall growth, development, and health maintenance. Lastly, when there are deficiencies within the identified essential requirements, it can lead to problems in the development for children and adolescents, increased risks of diseases in adults, and declining health in older adults. Health care providers should utilize published resources to assist individuals in choosing and maximizing nutrient-rich foods that support their current life cycle.

Physical activity is a constant factor in making personalized recommendations for individuals in the context of a nutritional assessment. Moreover, the connection between physical activity and weight management is well established and should be incorporated when possible. Physical activity is crucial for overall weight management through burning calories that could create a caloric deficit and increasing metabolism by increasing muscle mass [4]. Physiologically, exercise or physical activity has several metabolic effects throughout the body such as improving hormone regulation, enhancing mood, preserving lean mass, and stabilizing appetite [5]. The adaptations due to regular activity can be beneficial for weight management, weight loss, and overall health goals. Additional consideration should be given to the type and intensity of the exercise that will be used. Not everyone can tolerate high intensity aerobic (with oxygen or cardiovascular) activity for an extended period. Therefore, individuals should work with an exercise professional to find their mode of exercise and then determine the most effective way to incorporate the activity into their lifestyle [6]. The general recommendations of 30 minutes of aerobic activity per week can show modest changes in weight and body composition changes; however, for most individuals adding 150 minutes of moderate intensity or 75 minutes of vigorous activity with at least two days of strength training can provide the positive effects discussed above [7]. Bottom line is to get individuals moving and create consistency as this will help achieve long-term weight management that provides overall health benefits beyond just burning calories.

The last consideration for individuals when assessing their health status is paired up with physical activity as body composition goals can be intertwined. As previously discussed, the key components of fat mass (FM) and fat free mass (FFM) and the ratio are essential to understand as it relates to overall health. Higher visceral fat increases the risk of certain chronic diseases and metabolic health, therefore optimizing an individual's body composition that is needed. Individual's weight is a factor; however, the ratio of the FM to FFM is more important than weight alone. Increasing available active muscle tissue supports metabolism and strength while reducing excess fat. This creates an interesting paradigm where muscle tissue weighs more because the tissue is denser and more compact than fat tissue [8]. It can be frustrating for individuals to focus on a specific number on a scale as they are not losing weight, when in fact they are changing their body composition. Therefore, assessing the individuals FM/FFM ratio at the beginning of dietary and physical activity changes is essential. If there is excessive fat tissue to lose the initial weight, changes will be significant, and as the individual maintains dietary and physical activity, emphasis should be on the body composition changes rather than exclusive weight changes. This is an excellent motivation and tracking tool for individual goals which will be discussed in a later chapter.

Lifestyle Considerations and Personal Preferences

The next section in making nutrition-focused recommendations is the individual's specific lifestyle and personal preferences. Considerations of an individual's preferences focus on the personalization that generic advice and guidelines cannot provide. Some of this information could be collected during the initial health assessment or once an initial consultation has been done. Collecting information on access to food, food likes/dislikes, dietary habits, and goals can guide a conversation. More in-depth questions exploring activity levels, daily schedule, stress levels, and family/friend support can help understand the individual's environment to address where change can happen. There are areas to concentrate on to successfully address changes to become more sustainable as they align with their preferences.

Dietary preferences and restrictions Everyone will have unique dietary components that might include cultural traditions which might include the use of vegetarian/vegan diets or times of fasting to celebrate holidays or mark religious observances. General food likes/dislikes could include textures, taste (sweet/salty/umami), overall sensory appeal, and food habits. Considering factors such as these will help identify preferred healthy foods and possible suitable alternatives to ensure adherence to any dietary changes that might be made.

Budgetary or food access restrictions There are financial considerations and physical barriers to accessing food for some individuals. Food insecurity can affect all households and is not income dependent. Whether it is a financial limit due to balancing household needs (rent, utilities, or healthcare) or a physical barrier (lack of transportation or food desert) can impact food availability. With a reduced quality or variety of foods, it may result in lower total calories, deficiencies in macro- and micronutrients, and increased risk of chronic diseases [9]. Education on food assistance programs, food budgeting, and cooking skill development can help decrease food insecurity and improve nutrition-related health outcomes.

Lifestyle behaviors and routines Utilizing an individual's daily routine, work schedule, stress levels, and where meal planning fits into a daily life is important. These factors can influence the individual's food choices, adherence to dietary changes, metabolic health, and weight management. An analysis in this area can help individuals understand what food choices are important to them and where modifications could happen. Highlighting the importance of good sleep hygiene, lowering stress, incorporating physical activity, and establishing sustainable dietary changes can impact health. Making better food choices is sometimes difficult when there is an established habit within daily life. For example, skipping meals due to work schedule or lack of planning can be a hard habit to correct for some because it becomes embedded in daily life. Personalizing strategies that fit their life routines and education to support change will help make new behaviors and routines that support overall health.

Foundational Nutrition Education

A large area for consideration is nutrition-focused recommendations education piece. A health care provider could make suggestions and changes to an individual's dietary nutrition; however, if the individual does not understand the "why" for the recommendations, it will not be valuable. A good rule of thumb is to start small and keep it simple. Addressing their diet currently is common ground for opening the conversation about what could change. This will assess their understanding of the current diet, willingness to make change, and overall motivation. Through conversations health care providers will identify current habits, any nutrient gaps, and areas for improvement. This information can be gathered either through interviewing or using questionnaires.

Either way, it provides the information where changes can be made while assessing the foundational knowledge that may need to be improved upon. Therefore, empowering individuals with foundational knowledge about "why" certain foods are important for their daily life will increase their investment and involvement in making dietary changes. There are four areas of nutrition education that should be recommended and then tailored to the individual.

Focusing on natural foods There are ways to educate individuals here: focusing on plant-based, nutrient-dense foods, decreasing the amount of ultra-processed foods, reading nutrition labels, and learning how to make simple swaps.

1. Plant-based, nutrient-dense foods: Recommendations on increasing fruits, vegetables, whole grains, and lean proteins will ensure total calories and quality sources of vitamins, minerals, and fiber. By highlighting this concept, individuals can learn that these sources will give their body the essential pieces to lower the risk of chronic diseases and provide steady caloric energy support. Part of the education includes explaining benefits of "how" these foods support health. Concepts such as fiber aiding digestion and regulating blood sugar, complex carbohydrates helping preserve protein for synthesis, and a variety of plant-based foods reducing inflammation illustrate the 'how'.
2. Decreasing the amount of ultra-processed foods (UPFs): Limiting UPFs is important because research has shown increased risks for chronic diseases (type 2 diabetes, cardiovascular disease, metabolic disorders), disrupted gut health, and potential for addictive-like properties [10]. UPFs are typically lower in fiber, overprocessed which can strip essential vitamins and minerals, and contain additives which can disrupt the microbiome. Current climate of food distribution and processing makes it difficult to eliminate some level of processing in foods. However, educating individuals to identify UPFs in various foods and cut back on those items can help make dietary and health improvements.

3. Reading nutrition labels: This is one of the most underutilized, but important skills individuals can develop to help manage their diet. There are several educational websites, apps, and tools that can be used; however, teaching the basics is the most effective way. Here is quick step-by-step method to highlight the importance of reading labels.
    - Quick scan → calories per serving, single serving size, added sugars, and how many ingredients. What do these four points tell you about an item?
    - Find the macronutrients → what is the ratio of carbohydrates to protein to fat? What percentage of these meets the daily value? How much fiber is in the product?
    - Find the micronutrients → are the big vitamins and minerals in this product? Look for the essentials: vitamin D, calcium, iron, and potassium as they are required to be listed on food labels. What percentage of these meet the daily value?

    Keeping these concepts simple and consistent, individuals can quickly scan an item to see how worthy it is for their diet. Starting with an individual's favorite item like cereal or snack will make the concept relevant. You can also challenge individuals to compare and contrast or find the best option to incorporate into their diet.
4. Simple swaps: This technique can be another tool for individuals to reduce the intake of UPFs, additional sugars, and unhealthy fats. Simple exchanges to swap out less healthy ingredients with ones that are lower in calories, higher in fiber, and provide reliable sources of vitamins and minerals can improve the diet. Some common examples of swaps are:
    - Mayonnaise → hummus or mustard—still provides flavor with more fiber and less unhealthy fats.
    - Sugar in coffee → small amount of honey or maple sugar—reduces refined sugars and adds natural flavor.
    - Sour cream → Greek yogurt—still provides flavor and better source of protein with probiotics for the gut.

These four concepts highlight the educational tools for individuals to learn and implement into their diets. Combining information with opportunities to practice skills makes a significant impact on emphasizing why incorporating dietary choices impacts long-term health. Most importantly, these concepts can gradually be incorporated into daily practice without making immediate changes that might discourage individuals.

Calorie balance and management The concept of calories can be an elusive piece of nutritional education; it is no longer the simple saying of "calories in equals calories out." The old saying can be used as a guideline; however, the understanding goes beyond simple balance and is more about the management of calories. Breaking these concepts into individual areas will help see the importance of each as it pertains to the energy value of calories.

1. *Calorie balance*: In the simplest terms, calorie balance will determine if an individual gains, loses, or maintains weight. The balance between caloric intake (energy in) and caloric output (energy out) ensures that normal body functions can be maintained. To maintain their current weight, an individual must burn approximately the same number of calories that they consume each day. The weight gain scenario requires an individual to consume more calories than they are expending or the body would use. Finally, individuals would lose weight by creating a calorie deficit where less calories are consumed while calories expended through activity are greater. The caloric balance is a straightforward way to describe the relationship between calories in versus calories out. This is simplistic way to start conversations about calories, and the emphasis in practice would be to focus on the eating patterns. Combining a healthy diet that contains recommended nutrients in appropriate portions with physical activity can help create a healthy balance.

2. *Calorie management*: Once calorie balance is learned, it can help further explain the key aspects of calorie management. The practice of managing one's calories will take practice as it will require a deeper understanding of the nutrient's caloric quality. Focusing on the recommendation of nutrient-dense foods that increase fullness or satiety and affect metabolism is important. For example, foods that are protein rich and paired with a higher fiber source can boost satiety by slowing digestion. The combination of nutrient-dense sources can stabilize blood sugar, support metabolism, and reduce overall calorie intake [11]. Therefore, if an individual has two snacks in front of them that have equal overall calories, the quality or density of the one snack has greater worth nutritionally. Educating individuals that pre-packaged, processed food fails to provide better calorie fueling and the nutrients that the body needs is important. Additionally, there is another opportunity to use the simple swaps that would focus on the better quality, nutrient-dense choices of food or snacks. Overall, individuals that choose nutrient-dense options by swapping out processed or low-quality calorie foods can help manage their hunger levels and support the metabolism.

Calorie balance and management education is crucial for making recommendations to individuals as it will aid in providing the foundational knowledge for maintaining healthy body weight. Important distinctions between the balance and management of calories consumed will lead to informed decision-making for their diet. This shift optimizes individual nutrient intake; rather than focusing solely on total calories, individuals begin to recognize that the quality of those calories matters more.

Behavioral and Health Psychological Aspects

The final area to consider in the nutritional focused recommendations will be the behavioral and psychological aspects that will shape nutrition and health changes. Health care professionals will have two charges as they make their recommendations for dietary change, address the established behaviors and habits, and introduce new behavioral strategies to create change. Both charges are equally important as individuals will examine their motives, personality, beliefs, and attitudes toward food and nutrition. This process is unique to the individual and will help identify dietary areas to change, recognize barriers that might interfere with change, and develop skills and solutions to achieve nutrition-related goals.

Psychological factors influencing nutrition Individuals develop nutritional preferences from a combination of environment, genetics, and culture. Each of these preferences plays a role in directing our choices and behaviors around food. For example, the family environment can influence types of food eaten, loyalty to certain brands, traditions, and dislikes. This can be very influential at a subconscious level until an individual changes an environment and exposed to new food experiences. To understand these influences, it is important to look at the psychological factors that are considered [12].

1. *Self-efficacy and control*: An individual's confidence in their ability to make healthy food choices plays a leading role in nutrition. When individuals feel they have control over their eating habits, they are more likely to set realistic goals, resist temptations, and maintain long-term dietary changes. Without this sense of self-efficacy, even the best nutrition plans can fall apart.
2. *Emotion and mood*: Food and emotions are intertwined. Stress, anxiety, or depression often leads to comfort eating or avoiding meals altogether, while certain foods can directly influence mood through biochemical pathways. For example, sugar may provide a temporary boost but can worsen emotional lows later, creating a cycle that affects both mental health and nutrition.
3. *Cognitive biases*: The way individuals perceive health, body image, and food quality shapes their choices. Cognitive biases can lead to distorted eating patterns, such as orthorexia, where individuals become overly fixated on "clean" or "pure" foods. These mental shortcuts influence decisions about what is considered healthy, often pushing people toward extremes rather than balance.

4. *Habits and cravings*: Ultra-processed foods are engineered to stimulate dopamine pathways, making them highly addictive. Over time, these cravings form entrenched habits that are difficult to break, even when individuals consciously want to eat healthier. This explains why unhealthy eating patterns often persist despite awareness of their negative consequences.

Psychological influences on nutrition demonstrate that dietary behavior is not merely a matter of knowledge or access to food but is profoundly shaped by an individual's preferences. The personal preferences, often formed early and reinforced through repeated exposure, play a decisive role in shaping eating habits. Once established, these preferences can become deeply ingrained, making individuals resistant to change even when faced with addressing health issues.

Introducing new behavioral strategies Understanding the psychological factors that influence individual's dietary choices will help introduce new strategies and implement them in their daily lives. Long-term sustainability of dietary change depends on cultivating practical behavioral shifts that empower individuals to take ownership of their health. Education serves as a unifying theme, reinforcing these changes by encouraging greater awareness of eating habits and physical activity. Key strategies include practicing portion control, choosing nutrient-dense foods and healthy swaps, and tuning into hunger and satiety cues. As individuals assimilate nutritional knowledge into everyday routines, these behaviors become second nature. Learning how to make informed choices and decisions about their diets will ensure long-term success by maintaining a healthy weight and decreasing their risk of chronic diseases. Specific behavioral strategies utilized for making nutritional recommendations will include patient-centered approaches or multi-level interventions.

1. *Patient-centered approaches*: The approach will partner health care providers and the individual, possibly including family members, to explore perspectives, knowledge, and problem-

solving. This is a collaborative experience in which methods could include decision-making, meal planning, goal setting, and discussing how to prepare for potential barriers or nutritional adjustments. The approach will utilize foundational nutritional knowledge that the individual will use to make informed decisions and behavioral changes within their diet. The long-term effect for the individual will increase their cognitive skills to determine the best path toward achieving healthy behaviors and adherence to dietary changes.

2. *Multi-level Interventions*: One framework that works very well within the domain of health is the Social-Ecological Model (SEM). This model allows health care providers to develop interventions based on the interconnected levels between individual, interpersonal, organizational/community, and policy/societal factors [13]. The framework of the model can help identify an individual's dietary habits based on immediate impacts of the surrounding environment (personal factors, family, social network) and the broader, large-scale environment (politics, laws, cultural norms, and economic conditions) [14]. Examples of addressing the levels could include:
   (a) Individual—Increasing awareness of nutrient-dense foods through education and companion shopping.
   (b) Interpersonal—Cooking class with family to try new foods and meals.
   (c) Organizational/Community—Work with local agencies (YMCA, school, food banks) to offer reduced memberships, classes for families, or neighborhood events to promote physical activity and access to foods.
   (d) Policy/societal factors—Connecting patients with healthy food access (government programs for food assistance), fresh produce in community gardens, or access to telehealth professionals.

   The SEM provides a powerful framework for driving meaningful change by recognizing the multiple layers that shape an individual's daily life. It highlights how both immediate environmental factors and broader societal influences, often beyond personal control, interact to affect behavior and outcomes. By designing interventions that simultaneously address these interconnected levels, practitioners can create comprehensive strategies that not only foster individual growth but also generate wider educational and community impact.

Behavioral and psychological factors play a critical role in shaping nutrition and health outcomes. Effective dietary recommendations must address both established habits and the introduction of new behavioral strategies. Nutritional preferences are influenced by environment, genetics, and culture, with family traditions and early exposure often guiding food choices at a subconscious level. Recognizing these influences is essential for tailoring interventions that resonate with each individual's unique context. Sustainable dietary change depends on cultivating behavioral shifts supported by education and self-awareness. Strategies such as portion control, selecting nutrient-dense foods, making healthy swaps, and listening to hunger and satiety cues help individuals integrate nutritional knowledge into daily routines. Patient-centered approaches and multi-level interventions ensure that recommendations are both personalized and scalable, ultimately promoting long-term health, weight management, and reduced risk of chronic disease.

Chapter Summary

Developing effective nutrition-focused recommendations requires a multidimensional approach that integrates current recommendations, nutritional considerations, personal context, and health or behavioral psychology. Once the essential components of a nutritional assessment are assembled, the next step is to translate findings into personalized strategies that support individual goals. Macronutrient guidance must be tailored to the individual, considering lifestyle, preferences, and health status, while remaining aligned with current nutritional guidelines. Opportunities for establishing foundational nutrition education and addressing habits and/or attitudes that shape dietary decisions can empower individuals. Education reinforces these behavioral shifts by increasing awareness of eating habits and physical activity. Nutrition-focused recommendations are most effective when they combine patient-centered approaches with multi-level interventions. This ensures that nutrition recommendations are not only personalized but also scalable, creating a comprehensive framework for sustainable dietary change and improved health outcomes.

Chapter Review Questions

1. What are the four key areas that guide nutrition-focused recommendations, and how do they interact to create a personalized framework for dietary change?
2. How can psychological factors such as environment, genetics, and culture influence an individual's dietary choices, and what strategies can health professionals use to address these influences?
3. Why is education considered important in sustaining long-term dietary change, and how does it reinforce behavioral strategies such as portion control and hunger/satiety awareness?
4. The use of simple swaps in a diet can increase the overall nutrient density by replacing high-calorie, processed items. How would a health care provider educate individuals? Give an example of various foods or meals where a swap could be made.
5. Compare patient-centered approaches with multi-level interventions in nutrition counseling. What are the strengths and limitations of each in promoting sustainable health outcomes?

References

1. Dietaryguidelines.gov. https://www.dietaryguidelines.gov/sites/default/files/2020-12/Dietary_Guidelines_for_Americans_2020-2025.pdf
2. Gropper SS. The role of nutrition in chronic disease. Nutrients. 2023;15(3):664. https://doi.org/10.3390/nu15030664.
3. Faizan U, Rouster AS. Nutrition and hydration requirements in children and adults. In: StatPearls. Treasure Island: StatPearls Publishing; 2025.
4. Kadam SJ. Weight management and various other benefits of physical activity in human life. Eur J Sport Sci. 2025;4(2):12–7. https://www.ej-sport.org/index.php/sport/article/view/223

5. Alyafei A, Balfour J, Keyes D. Physical activity and weight loss maintenance. In: StatPearls. Treasure Island: StatPearls Publishing; 2025.
6. Arney BE, Glover R, Fusco A, Cortis C, de Koning JJ, van Erp T, et al. Comparison of RPE (rating of perceived exertion) scales for session RPE. Int J Sports Physiol Perform. 2019;14(7):994–6. https://doi.org/10.1123/ijspp.2018-0637.
7. Jayedi A, Soltani S, Emadi A, Zargar M-S, Najafi A. Aerobic exercise and weight loss in adults: A systematic review and dose-response meta-analysis: A systematic review and dose-response meta-analysis. JAMA Netw Open. 2024;7(12):e2452185. https://doi.org/10.1001/jamanetworkopen.2024.52185.
8. Park J, Kim S. Validity of muscle-to-fat ratio as a predictor of adult metabolic syndrome. J Phys Ther Sci. 2016;28(3):1036–45. https://doi.org/10.1589/jpts.28.1036.
9. Wetherill MS, White KC, Rivera C. Food insecurity and the nutrition care process: Practical applications for dietetics practitioners. J Acad Nutr Diet. 2018;118(12):2223–34. https://doi.org/10.1016/j.jand.2017.08.114.
10. Rondinella D, Raoul PC, Valeriani E, Venturini I, Cintoni M, Severino A, et al. The detrimental impact of ultra-processed foods on the human gut microbiome and gut barrier. Nutrients. 2025;17(5):859. https://doi.org/10.3390/nu17050859.
11. Njike VY, Smith TM, Shuval O, Shuval K, Edshteyn I, Kalantari V, et al. Snack food, satiety, and weight. Adv Nutr. 2016;7(5):866–78. https://doi.org/10.3945/an.115.009340.
12. Hardcastle SJ, Thøgersen-Ntoumani C, Chatzisarantis NLD. Food choice and nutrition: a social psychological perspective. Nutrients. 2015;7(10):8712–5. https://doi.org/10.3390/nu7105424.
13. Oudat Q, Okour A. Utilizing the Social Ecological Model to inform nursing practice for improved childhood eating behaviors. Res Theory Nurs Pract. 2025;39(3):319–30. https://doi.org/10.1891/RTNP-2024-0169.
14. Ecological models of behavior change. Change Theories Collection. 2022. https://ascnhighered.org/ASCN/change_theories/collection/ecological_models.html

Goal Setting 8

Abstract

Goal setting plays a central role in translating nutritional assessment data into personalized strategies for meaningful behavior change. As a foundational psychological practice, goal setting provides individuals with direction, structure, and motivation as they work to modify dietary and activity habits. This chapter examines the elements of effective goal pursuit, including the distinction between nutritional goals and body-weight-focused goals, the use of intrinsic and extrinsic rewards, and the development of short- and long-term goals. It also explores the evolution of goal-setting theory and the role of habit formation, highlighting both traditional goal-based approaches and identity-based strategies. By understanding how to connect intention to action, individuals and practitioners can create sustainable pathways toward improved health behaviors and long-term success.

Keywords

Goal setting · Behavior change · Habit formation · Intrinsic and extrinsic rewards · Short- and long-term goals · Goal pursuit Motivation

S. Kitts, *Nutritional Assessment*,
https://doi.org/10.1007/978-3-032-22506-1_8

Learning Objectives:
By the end of this chapter, students should be able to:

- Explain the role of goal setting in nutritional assessment and behavior change.
- Differentiate between nutritional goals and body-weight-focused goals.
- Compare intrinsic and extrinsic rewards and their influence on sustaining behavior change.
- Develop short- and long-term goals that support dietary and activity improvements.
- Analyze how habit formation—both goal-based and identity-based—supports long-term behavior change.

The use of goal setting in nutritional assessment is the critical step where the assessment data can be used to build individual strategies for success. Goal setting has been established as a fundamental psychological skill or practice that can provide a direction for individuals to manage change daily. Additionally, goal setting gives individuals a framework to facilitate behavior change in an area that they deem changes need to be made. The framework can include enhancing motivation, providing focus, and monitoring progress as the individual makes changes to build consistent, healthy habits. Fundamentally, psychology describes goals for individuals as a desired future state that will be supported by preceding events that help to meet the end state [1]. However, achieving goals can be difficult because the individual must find a way to connect intention to action to be successful. Educating individuals on how to implement change through goal setting will support steps to make lasting dietary and activity improvements. This chapter will review the elements of goal pursuit, the concepts or methods utilized, habit formation, and strategies for lasting change.

Goal Setting in Nutritional Assessment

The use of goal setting is universal for the general population; using specifically in the nutritional assessment will enhance the individual's experience. Health care providers can emphasize the importance of identifying individual's needs, collaborate with goal setting, and bridge the gap between clinical recommendations and personal preferences. An example of this is the difference between nutritional goals and body weight goals.

Nutritional goals Individuals might need guidance when setting goals for their nutrition because they might not understand current concepts or recommendations. Health care providers can help here by focusing on improving the overall quality of the diet and nutrients by educating them on small changes that can be made to the current diet. For example, an individual might put a goal of eating better but not knowing how to do practically do this. Better goals could be to reduce eating processed foods three times a week or increase fiber content by incorporating fruits and vegetables at each meal. These are behavior-focused and qualitative targets for individuals to achieve.

Body weight goals There are several individual factors that may play into setting body weight goals. Unlike nutritional goals, the focus may center on a particular number but not account for body composition or health conditions. The nutritional assessment will gather appropriate data from body mass index (BMI), body composition or difference between muscle and fat tissue, and specific individual factors. Health care providers should educate individuals on setting realistic weight goals that will promote the overall quality of life. For example, if an individual is obese, losing weight and changing their BMI can improve overall health. Goals can focus on quantitative, outcome-focused goals that will reduce weight and maintain muscle mass.

The relationship between these goals becomes interrelated once the nutritional assessment reveals what will need to be addressed. Only addressing one of the goals without the other will not provide a holistic plan to address the individual's needs. Weight goals without nutrition goals could lead to weight loss due to lack of total calories or essential nutrients. This is not an ideal method of losing weight as nutrition can support individual weight loss. Therefore, nutrition goals can support weight loss as healthy eating behaviors that account for total calories, higher fiber, and appropriate protein will support sustainable weight loss. Concepts like these will help health care providers develop individual-centered goals.

Elements of Goal Pursuit

There are essential elements that should be considered when preparing to set and reach goals. These elements can vary from source to source; therefore, the most common fundamental strategies will be discussed. A key principle to keep in mind moving forward is individual focus and simplicity.

Identifying a priority goal Most individuals will fall into two categories when identifying a goal; broad that will change to many things at once or too narrow an idea that cannot be supported. Conversations about a priority goal should first focus on the "what" do they want to change? A well-defined goal should reflect their personal intent to make changes and the time they can give this goal. Additionally, what is the reason or driving force to meet this goal? This process will help to decide the actions that will be put in place to achieve the goal in an effective way. Brainstorming a group of actions before any action happens will fully develop a goal and greater success of reaching the goal.

Creating specific action Once an individual has identified the priority goal and started examining the actions that will be taken, a more specific plan is developed. The focus in this area is the "how" the actions will be prioritized and managed. One way to do this is using goal setting models that will help to determine which actions are needed and for how long it takes to reach the goal. Models for goal setting will be discussed in detail in this chapter; however, the essential pieces include assigning resources if needed, setting and adjusting timelines, and assessment of actions. This is aided by using short-term and long-term goals as it allows individuals to regularly review progress and reflect on goals that will need to be adjusted. This is called an action-orientated plan; individuals focus on more specific details and narrow the purpose of making these changes.

Measuring and assessing goals This action step can be done in several different ways, and the individual should determine the way that will keep them accountable. Using short-term goals, an individual can track progress by breaking down information and documenting. Using a calendar, journal, or mobile apps will help to show changes and increase adherence to the individual. Tracking progress can be done by recording physical measurements such as weight and girth measurements, noting visual progress, and performance metrics like activity logs. Practices like these can boost motivation and align efforts with the individuals' goal objectives [2]. The use of behavioral measures such as fitness wearables, dietary journaling, and measuring physical activity is very useful.

Flexibility and adaptability of goals The ability to compare individual's perceived reality to the end goal is an essential piece of goal setting. Feedback and evaluation of the actions will move individuals closer to their target as they reach a milestone. This feedback also provides information on potential roadblocks that might slow or hinder their movement toward the goal. This is where flexibility and adaptation of smaller goals or actions can be modified. The focus here can be "why" an action wasn't completed or stopped them from being successful? Instances like these are a chance to reassess and modify an action so that success can continue. It can be frustrating; however, education and emphasis should be placed on reframing from the setback, learning, and focusing on the consistency of the action. Embracing setbacks as learning opportunities will foster the ability to see future setbacks and how to manage them.

Intermittent Rewards Goal setting can foster sustainable change by reinforcing positive behaviors or rewards. There are two different kinds of rewards—intrinsic and extrinsic rewards—that can be sources of motivation for individuals. Intrinsic rewards are important as they come from the internal satisfaction of accomplishment. The sense of autonomy gained from an activity based on the individual's preference or interest drives long-term engagement [3]. For example, an individual who makes dietary changes and sees their total cholesterol decrease is more likely to continue making healthier choices. The individual values the changes they have made to their diet and will commit to the process.

Extrinsic rewards come from the external environment and some materialistic sources. Motivation is not driven by the activity, rather the reward like praise from others, avoidance of negative consequences, or tangible benefits [3]. The external reward is deriving satisfaction instead of the accomplishment of the activity. For example, an individual joins a gym weight loss challenge to win gift cards but doesn't continue activity after the challenge. Compared to intrinsic, extrinsic rewards lead to short-term success and may not transfer to long-term engagement.

Intrinsic and extrinsic rewards can be used to motivate individuals; however, the best kind of motivation may vary depending on situation and individual preferences. Combining extrinsic goals to intrinsic values can be complementary [3]. Implementing small extrinsic rewards for milestones toward the priority goal is beneficial in positive associations. Ultimately, goal setting that include engagement and incentives will reinforce behaviors in making healthy choices.

Health care providers will act as guides by using these fundamental elements in goal pursuit for individuals. Education for individuals will define their goals and achieve personalized, sustainable goals that will motivate them to make changes. The nutritional assessment will move the data from a supportive role by bridging the individual goals to engage in efforts.

Review of Goal Setting Methods

The fundamental elements of goal setting have evolved with time to keep pace with the needs of individuals in current times. Historically, philosophers and psychologists recognized that giving a purpose to an action can help individuals increase drive to accomplish goals. The ability to link specific tasks to challenge individuals and receive feedback laid out the foundation for contemporary goal setting, framework, and theories. The following highlighted goal setting techniques will help bring structure to the individual's overall goals. However, the essential inclusion and use of short- and long-term goals will create the foundation for improvement.

Short-term goals The use of short-term goals is essential and depends on the complexity of the long-term goal. Short-term goals are seen as process-orientated and will help provide clarity and focus for breaking down the end point into manageable pieces. Additionally, assigning a time factor to short-term goals can provide momentum, motivation, and feedback on the individual's progress. Managing two to five short-term goals is a general guideline, as too many will make it difficult or overwhelming for the individual. Therefore, once the individual has a long-term goal, it can be broken down into smaller, actionable steps with a clear process. The process should include measurable steps that include a reasonable time frame. Having these steps will provide a distinct milestone that is directly related to the end goal. Once a short-term goal is achieved, assessment of the feedback and actions that were met will need to be re-examined and modified to continue to move toward the end goal. Setting new short-term goals shows accomplishment toward health goals.

Long-term goal(s) The overarching goal for an individual will give meaning to the daily efforts and provide direction, assessment, and management of the short-term goal process. Long-term goals are outcome-oriented goals, meaning that focus is placed on the final, tangible results rather than daily actions. Unlike short-term goals which are considered the "how" or process, long-term goals are the "what" or outcomes of the summative process. The time frame here may exceed months or a year depending on the goal and time to achieve. For individuals, determining the importance of a long-term goal over time will also enhance decision-making and help prioritize their efforts and action that align with the outcome. Typically, individuals will pick one long-term goal, supported by the short-term goals that can be modified once they are complete. This will foster individual growth, self-confidence, and satisfaction that goals can be achieved.

An example of an individual that wants to work toward lowering high cholesterol and sodium through dietary changes is as follows:

Long-term goal: (Time frame: 6 months) Make manageable changes that reduce saturated fats, added sodium, and processed foods.

Short-term goal: (Time frame: 4 weeks)

- Swap high-sodium convenience foods (canned soups, frozen meals, deli meats) for lower-sodium options or homemade versions.
- Add one serving of soluble-fiber foods daily (oats, beans, lentils, apples) to help lower LDL cholesterol.
- Cook more meals at home using herbs, citrus, and spices instead of salt for flavor.

Outcome: Early reductions in sodium intake and saturated fat, slight improvements in cholesterol levels, and increased awareness of food choices.

In this example, the individual can keep a journal to record the changes they have made to visualize progress. Additionally, continued education and use of mobile apps to scan items purchased or find healthier recipes can be tracked. These steps will help individuals meet long-term nutritional goals and possibly make lifestyle, sustainable changes.

Review of Established Goal Setting Methods

Once the short- and long-term goals are defined, the next task will be to determine a method or framework to give structure and understanding to the individual. There are several different methods or frameworks that have been used, and the review of three established methods will be discussed. The most cohesive approach for the individual should be the focus, and health care providers should help to determine the best approach for each case.

Early Goal-Setting Theory

In the 1970s and 1980s, the foundational basis began for later renditions of goal setting with the help of the work done by Locke's Goal-Setting Theory. The theory states that if an individual has specific and challenging goals, it will in turn motivate and increase their performance [4]. The key principles of clarity, challenge, commitment, feedback, and task complexity will focus on the individual by increasing effort to reach the goal through persistence. The advantage of Locke's theory can be applied to individuals, teams, and performance goals in professional settings. The multiple sites this theory can be utilized will set clear direction, increased motivation, reach performance highs, and help set specific goals that can provide feedback. There are disadvantages as well; individuals who have used this theory cite a tendency toward tunnel vision due to highly specific goals, a lack of flexibility within rigid structures, and limited use of available resources to support goal achievement [4]. Ultimately, Locke's theory shows the relationship between conscious goals and achievement. If an individual sets a vague or less detailed goal, they may encounter lower motivation and goal achievement. Therefore, set challenging goals that will motivate individuals to actively pursue improvement and performance.

Applying Locke's theory in health and nutrition is appropriate as it can direct focus on relevant actions like choosing whole grains over ultra-processed breads. Health care providers can help with reframing vague goals to enhance clarity and specificity for individuals. For example, if an individual wants to "lose weight," they will need to focus on how to achieve this by stating "eating 250 fewer calories and moving for 20 minutes a day will help with weight loss in the next four months." This creates a personal buy-in to manage overall calories and make sustainable choices to achieve the goal. Statements like this remove the vague weight loss by adding a process goal that will need the individual to focus on the execution of certain behaviors.

SMART Goals

In 1981, Doran presented a structured framework that highlighted Locke's managing goals through emphasizing clarity and applying measurability [5]. Doran applied an acronym SMART—Specific, Measurable, Attainable/Achievable/Assignable, Realistic, Time bound. This type of framework gives individuals a clear understanding of the direction they will need to take to achieve their goal. An example of each part can be found below; this shows the ownership over the goal-setting process.

Specific—What do I want to achieve and how will I achieve this goal?
Measurable—How will I track feedback and success in accomplishing the goal?
Achievable—Do I have the resources or support to achieve this goal?
Realistic—Will the goal align with my overall goals?
Time bound—What are the milestones and deadline for this goal?

The SMART framework can also be applied to nutrition goals by removing vague statements and exchanging them with clear goals that will focus on the broader health outcomes. Using the framework to write a personal statement that would encompass the acronym can be impactful. For example, "I will plan and pack lunches everyday (specific, measurable, realistic) for the entire month (time bound) to eat at work to control intake of calories and sodium (relevant, achievable)." Statements like these increase the likelihood of success by focusing on progress, allowing feedback, and adjusting when needed. The coordination of health care providers and patient-centric goals with this framework can make measurable strides to improve overall health outcomes.

SMARTER Framework

Finally, in 2016, Hyatt extended the earlier goal setting frameworks by adding the "ER" or Exciting/ Evaluated and Risk/Revised pieces. The addition of the last two items to the acronym attempted to make the goal-setting application more practical and include the individual mindset. The idea was to include actionable verbs that could be linked to goals and the habits that are present [6]. This is an interesting modification that individuals can consider as linking the goals to consistent daily or weekly habits is crucial for clarity and commitment. Although there has not been research to support the additions, for some individuals the realization of risk or excitement to reach the goal could be beneficial. Another caveat is direct accountability to the individual as they are encouraged to write down or share their goals with trusted individuals. An example of adding "ER" could be added to the previous SMART example; "I will plan and pack lunches everyday (specific, measurable, realistic) for the entire month (time bound) to eat at work to control intake of calories and sodium (relevant, achievable). After four weeks I will meet with the nutritionist (evaluated) to decide the next steps based on daily energy perception (revised)." This may make the personal statement longer; however, the additions highlight the accountability and evolution of the goal.

Key Takeaways on Goal-Setting Framework

The total evolution of goal setting ensures that individuals will have a framework to support meaningful and sustainable change. The earliest framework or theories focused on challenging goals to increase motivation with a lack of support or feedback for some individuals. By incorporating strategies and skills, an individual can use adjusted focus to learning the process rather than the outcome solely. Finally, specific adaptations from feedback offer a clearer picture of habits that can be linked to the goal. There is a middle ground between vague goals that might not produce change and challenging goals that can become overwhelming. Health care providers and individuals can therefore tailor the goals based on the individual needs, support, and feedback of the process.

Habit Formation

An underlying piece of information in goal setting is the connection to habits. The development of a habit can be inherently hard to change or modify because the brain builds strong neural pathways for repeated activities or automatic. Research has shown that these pathways can manifest comfort, gratification, and emotional triggers in a situation [7]. The neurobiology goes beyond the scope of this text; however, understanding that habits are ingrained in a neural system that will seek short-term rewards over possible long-term benefits is the foundation. For an individual to break a habit means fighting against the established neural pathways which will require significant effort and time to then establish a new habit.

Developing Habit Formation

There is a vast debate about how long it takes to form a habit so that it becomes automatic. A quick search online will yield a plethora of estimates; the general reported range is 18 to 254 days with the average of 66 days to create an automatic habit [8]. Individual variance is important to account for as some habits are more complex or the connection to making the change in habits will require more adherence from the individual. Health care providers can help individuals be successful by stressing that habit formation is about consistency over time, not perfection each day. Additionally, if a new behavior can be connected to the individual's current routine and behaviors, they are more likely to be incorporated. For example, the individual works out three times a week before work and they want to create a habit of not purchasing fast-food breakfast on the way to work. Instead, they brainstorm options that the individual can prep the night before and pack for themselves. This is a great way to support the already established activity habit and pair it with a nutritional habit that is easy to implement.

Parallel to goal pursuit and the use of intrinsic and extrinsic rewards, habits can be goal-based or identity based. These concepts offer a different approach for individuals to consider when starting to build habits that will support their outcomes. An overall goal of losing weight would be considered a goal-based habit. In contrast, an identity-based habit statement could be "I am someone who nourishes and moves my body to maintain health." This is a positive statement to not tie weight loss to a number on a scale while focusing on overall health. This shift in tone supports small, daily habits; actions like taking a 10–15 minute walk after dinner reinforce the desired identity without feeling overwhelming. The concept of identity-based habits can be powerful as it connects a habit to identity and creates internal motivation. Here is another example of how this can be written down for the individual to see the impact of habit change.

Identity: "I'm the kind of person who prioritizes my health."

Habit: Each morning, I pack a lunch with whole foods because that's what I prioritize for my health. In the evening, I take a short walk because movement is part of who I am. When I choose snacks, I pause and pick options that support my energy because that aligns with my identity.

Result: The focus isn't on losing weight—it's on living as the person I believe myself to be. Weight-related changes become a by-product of consistent identity-aligned actions.

The key take-away points for health care providers and individuals to consider are defining who they want to be, starting with small daily actions that support the habit, reflect on success, and reinforce the individual's identity. Habit formation can automate behaviors as action from the conscious effort to the subconscious streamlines the process [9]. The repetition of guided actions supports health behavior change directly through the individuals' desire for change. Therefore, health care providers and individuals should design the environment to implement actions and plan for unwanted habits when faced with them. Again, focusing on the process, not just the outcome, will help individuals implement an alternative response and keep moving forward on achieving an automation of the new habit [8].

Chapter Summary

The essential role of goal setting within nutritional assessment and behavior change is an important piece of the health outcome puzzle. Once assessment data are collected, goal setting becomes the pivotal step that transforms information into individualized strategies for success. As a well-established psychological practice, goal setting provides individuals with direction, structure, and a sense of purpose as they work to modify daily habits. It offers a framework that enhances motivation, sharpens focus, and supports ongoing progress monitoring. These are key components in developing consistent, health-promoting behaviors. Yet the process of achieving goals is often challenging, as individuals must bridge the gap between intention and action. Teaching individuals how to implement change through effective goal-setting practices can strengthen their ability to make lasting improvements in dietary patterns and physical activity.

This chapter explores the core elements of goal pursuit, including the distinction between nutritional goals and body-weight-focused goals, and the importance of aligning goals with meaningful personal outcomes. It reviews established goal-setting methods, such as short- and long-term goal development, and discusses how intermittent rewards, both intrinsic and extrinsic, can reinforce progress. The evolution of goal-setting theory and the role of habit formation, whether through traditional goal-based approaches or identity-based strategies, reshape how individuals view themselves and the ability to make change. These concepts provide a comprehensive foundation for understanding how goal setting can be used to support sustainable, individualized changes in nutrition and health behaviors.

Chapter Review Questions

1. Why is goal setting considered a critical step in translating nutritional assessment data into individualized strategies for change?
2. How do nutritional goals differ from body-weight-focused goals, and why is this distinction important for long-term success?
3. In what ways can intrinsic and extrinsic rewards influence an individual's progress toward their goals?
4. How do short-term and long-term goals work together to support sustainable dietary and activity changes?
5. What is the difference between goal-based habit formation and identity-based habit formation, and how might each approach benefit individuals seeking lasting change?

References

1. Berkman ET. The neuroscience of goals and behavior change. Consult Psychol J. 2018;70(1):28–44. https://doi.org/10.1037/cpb0000094.
2. Brusseau M, Gallet-Suchet B, Dray G, Gendrault S, Harguem L, Boiché J. Motivation toward physical activity and nutrition in older cancer patients: the MONAGE protocol using ecological momentary assessment and accelerometers. BMC Geriatr. 2025;25(1):431. https://doi.org/10.1186/s12877-025-06130-1.

3. Kumar P. Intrinsic vs. extrinsic motivation: What fuels our actions?. Psychology Town. 2024. Available from: https://psychology.town/motivation-emotion/intrinsic-vs-extrinsic-motivation-fuels-actions/
4. Locke EA, Latham GP. Building a practically useful theory of goal setting and task motivation. A 35-year odyssey. Am Psychol. 2002;57(9):705–17. Available from: https://med.stanford.edu/content/dam/sm/s-spire/documents/PD.locke-and-latham-retrospective_Paper.pdf
5. Bjerke MB, Renger R. Being smart about writing SMART objectives. Eval Program Plann. 2017;61:125–7. https://doi.org/10.1016/j.evalprogplan.2016.12.009.
6. Winter J. Mapping your path to success: The five pillars of goal-setting. Jeff Winter. 2024. Available from: https://www.jeffwinterinsights.com/insights/goal-setting-theory
7. Alexander R, Aragón OR, Bookwala J, Cherbuin N, Gatt JM, Kahrilas IJ, et al. The neuroscience of positive emotions and affect: Implications for cultivating happiness and wellbeing. Neurosci Biobehav Rev. 2021;121:220–49. https://doi.org/10.1016/j.neubiorev.2020.12.002.
8. Lally P, Gardner B. Promoting habit formation. Health Psychol Rev. 2013;7(sup1):S137–58. Available from: https://www.cykelvaeksthuset.dk/media/az3linp0/promoting-habit-formation.pdf
9. Gardner B, Lally P, Wardle J. Making health habitual: the psychology of "habit-formation" and general practice. Br J Gen Pract. 2012;62(605):664–6. https://doi.org/10.3399/bjgp12X659466.

Current Trends and Assessment Methods

9

Abstract

Advancements in digital health technologies are reshaping the way nutrition professionals assess dietary behaviors, metabolic responses, and overall health. This chapter examines how mobile applications, wearable devices, physiological sensors, continuous glucose monitors (CGMs), immersive virtual reality tools such as IVAN, and advanced biomarker testing enhance the precision and personalization of nutritional assessment. By integrating real-time data, behavioral insights, and biological indicators, these technologies support individualized dietary strategies that move beyond generalized recommendations. The chapter highlights how technology-driven assessment improves monitoring, supports behavior change, and enables more responsive, evidence-based nutrition interventions.

Keywords

Technology · Artificial intelligence · Mobile applications (apps) Mechanical sensor · Physiological sensor · Virtual reality "Omic" science · Biomarkers

S. Kitts, *Nutritional Assessment*,
https://doi.org/10.1007/978-3-032-22506-1_9

Learning Objectives:
By the end of this chapter, students should be able to:

- Explain how technology-based tools such as mobile apps, wearables, CGMs, and physiological sensors contribute to modern nutritional assessment.
- Differentiate between traditional assessment methods and advanced biomarker testing, including molecular tools and biological characteristic analysis.
- Evaluate how technology-generated data can be used to individualize dietary recommendations and health interventions.
- Discuss the benefits and limitations of integrating technology into nutrition practices.

Nutritional assessment has developed over the years to match population health trends, changing diet requirements, and overall lifestyle. Although the key foundational pieces remain, technology is moving the possibilities of assessment forward. Current nutrition trends focus on personalized and targeted nutrition, gut health, healthy aging, and accessible options, while assessment methods are becoming more advanced through technology like artificial intelligence (AI) for dietary analysis and wearables, alongside traditional methods like the ABCD approach (Anthropometric, Biochemical, Clinical, and Dietary). Other advanced techniques include metabolomics, nutrigenomics, and noninvasive methods like using dried blood spots to improve accuracy and accessibility.

Technology-Driven Assessment

Technology has changed so many things in our daily lives; it only makes sense that dietary assessment tools can be utilized and enhance dietary choices. The advancement of technology has improved health outcomes through the convenience of smartphones, tablets, wearables for tracking, apps, and artificial intelligence (AI). Accessible technology can streamline education and access information. Health care professionals can utilize various technologies to help individuals navigate the best ones to support their knowledge. The growing use of technology can improve accuracy and efficiency of disseminating knowledge, further education, and application. Additionally, researchers can also benefit from technological advancements by collecting large sets of data, offering virtual labs, globally collaborating on health issues, and analyzing behaviors. For these purposes, technology can incorporate established nutritional assessment into the real world through accessibility daily.

Mobile Applications (Apps)

Software programs that can be found on smartphones and tablets are categorized as a mobile app. There are a wider range of uses; however, they can provide an integration of specific information to the user. There are personalization components that the user can set up to help track activity or food calories, monitor health metrics like heart rate or sleep, and scan foods to determine the nutrient density. These apps can tailor content and provide feedback in real time. Individuals can use diet apps to record daily food intakes that can further be broken down into total calories, macronutrient distribution, and daily value of micronutrients. All this information can be compared to recommended guidelines and calculate goals for the individual. Dietitians that utilize apps with individuals recommend that these dietary tracking tools should be used as a guideline and supplement knowledge as there are some limitations [1]. Validity and reliability of the apps can lead to inconsistencies as they might underestimate calories and nutrient intakes. Individuals and health care providers can discuss the limitations to increase awareness on the consistency of apps to find the one that will work best. Overall, the use of dietary apps can promote consistency, increase self-monitoring, and enhance awareness of dietary choices [2].

Technology will continue to develop apps to support other aspects of an individual's dietary choices. Apps that can scan barcodes or take pictures of food will help to determine quality of foods, portion sizes, and amount of food processing. Current apps utilize research-based insights on nutritional quality scores, ultra-processed food classification, and detailed ingredient analysis. The apps can also highlight the environmental impact of food choices, giving users a broader understanding of how their food choices affect both health and sustainability. Apps like these are valuable to individuals that are invested in making dietary choices that will impact their daily lives.

Wearable Devices

Another area where technology has advanced tracking of health is found through wearable devices, watches, rings, and sensors. The wide range of devices now available has made it possible for everyone, from the general population to high-performing athletes, to track activity, calories burned, heart rate, and changes in body temperature. These devices are beneficial for increasing motivation and adherence to new health programming. The devices can be categorized into two types, movement sensors and physiological sensors.

- *Movement sensors*
  - *Pedometers:* The most common device that records individual steps throughout the day while wearing the device. The wearable pedometers today use accelerometers that will measure individual's movement in various directions and can detect speed changes too [3]. There are several smartwatches that have an incorporated pedometer which can make step counting and easy gauge for individuals to set a daily goal and monitor their progress. Health care providers have found that these devices increase the likelihood of step count adherence to promote active lifestyle changes in all age groups and those individuals seeking weight management strategies [3]. Other information that can be gathered with some devices is the conversion of the step count to distance covered. Calibrating a stride length through the

device will provide another way to track overall movement in an estimation of distance. For individuals that may not be able to work out every day, a simple understanding of averaging 2000 to 2500 equals steps per mile and equals about 20 minutes of activity [4]. This is a great opportunity to understand the importance of movement, reducing the risk of chronic diseases.

Accuracy of smartwatch pedometers is generally accurate for the general population and general daily use. This indicates that individuals that are tracking simple metrics like step counts and distance are good for motivating activity. These devices are less accurate for higher intensity activities or more complex data collection; consideration of activity level and brand/model will need to be considered for the individual.

– *Accelerometers/Gyroscopes*: These devices that include accelerometers and gyroscopes will enhance step counting and distance by accounting for the total volume of the activity and intensity. Devices that contain these will contain microelectromechanical systems (MEMS) which will utilize multiple sensors to capture more data such as heart rate, caloric expenditure, intensity level, and even sleep [3]. The accessibility of this technology in a smartwatch allows for more accurate reporting of athletic movements that are higher in intensity and specific movements found in various sports like swimming, cycling, and running. Additionally, some of these devices add global positioning satellite (GPS) information that can be used to monitor speed of an activity in real time, altitude, and pace. These smartwatches provide enough data to modify training and improve performance for individuals [3].

  Accuracy for these devices will track and collect data that is more specific to activity tracking that requires higher intensity or specific movements in various sports. The combination of accelerometer and gyroscopes technology has maintained less than 12% error regardless of gait or activity [5]. As technology advances, the sensor's ability to collect more data will also improve accuracy in determining the individual's effort over a wider range of activities.

- *Physiological Sensors*
  - *Heart rate monitoring:* This physiological sensor encompasses the standard heart rate monitors that require transducer pads to the smartwatch and chest strap devices. The non-medical devices that are worn across chest and pair with smartwatches have become a great method of monitoring individual athletes to a complete team during workouts. The device can monitor exercise intensity through the linear relationship between heart rate and VO_2 [3]. In exercise science, VO_2 max is the maximum (max) volume (V) measurement of oxygen (O_2) the body will utilize during intense exercise, making it a key metric for assessing cardiorespiratory fitness [6]. Devices such as these are useful in determining physiological changes that may occur in training and competition, metabolic demands during activity, and estimating energy needs.

    Accuracy for heart rate monitors that utilize a chest strap to collect data are considered the gold standard in higher intensity activities [7]. Brand and device models remain a factor for individuals to consider; however, the direct measurements of the heart electrical signals will provide more reliable data.
  - *Ring sensors:* This device is a newer way to monitor vital signs, activity, sleep patterns, and stress management. The technology in these devices relies on multiple sensors that include photoplethysmography (PPG), thermistors (skin temperature changes), and electrodermal activity (EDA) [8]. With the compact nature of the rings and user friendliness to connect to smartphones, users can monitor several health aspects in real time.

    Accuracy of the ring sensors remains to be seen as research has reported mixed results [8]. Much like other sensors, these rings should be used for general monitoring to provide insight into daily activity, calories burned, and biometrics such as sleep stages, heart rate, and VO_2max.

The advantages of wearables lie in improved technology, making it cost-effective and practical for people. Tracking real-time information provides individuals with feedback that they can use to increase their activity at work by getting up and moving or adjusting intensity levels of a workout. The increased awareness for the users will gain can help to bridge the gap between developing health goals and making them actionable outcomes. With time and continued technological advancements, the reliability will also advance.

Continuous Glucose Monitors (CGMs)

Technology to help track glucose levels in diabetic individuals has greatly improved from having multiple finger-stick to skin sensors that can be prescribed and/or over-the-counter (OTC) options. CGMs sensors will constantly monitor blood sugar levels and can help identify highs (hyperglycemia) or lows (hypoglycemia) in type 1 or type 2 diabetes. For individuals that may need to closely monitor their blood sugar levels daily and not using insulin, CGM can be a great management tool. The monitors can provide immediate information on the impact of diet and exercise, stress, and sleep on an individual's glucose response. This is an impactful educational tool as users will identify patterns like eating certain foods or exercise that can lead to better choices or meal timing. Moreover, diabetic individuals report that feedback that is gained through the CGMs increases motivation and adjusting decisions about their diet and/or exercise daily [9].

Technological advancements for pre- or diabetic individuals have enabled users to more actively manage their health. Monitors have been made to integrate with apps which can give visual feedback on their decisions and the impact on glucose levels. This information can also be shared with health care providers when there are questions or concerns about them from the users. CGMs have acceptable overall accuracy and reliability for the diabetic population for daily use. The key findings of CGMs should convey to users that individual differences, rapid glucose changes, and time lags due to ingestion will influence overall validity and consistency of readings [10]. Overall, this technological advancement has been well received and is a valuable tool for daily management of diabetes.

Interestingly, the introduction of OTC options has also opened the door to the general population using these monitors for general wellness. Individuals using CGMs that do not have a prediabetic or diabetic diagnosis are not necessarily needed. Currently there are no guidelines for non-diabetic individuals to use CGMs and could carry risks like anxiety or obsession with data, unhealthy diet choices, and misinterpretation of data that is collected [11]. If an individual has identifiable risk factors to be prediabetic or diabetic, there could be benefits through education as previously discussed. However, healthy individuals that are using CGMs to monitor normal blood sugar changes due to eating or exercising may be anecdotally interpreting data without medical context [11]. Healthy individuals may choose to use a CGM temporarily to understand the changes that can happen after eating or exercising, and it should not be used for an extended period. There are no guidelines or evidence for healthy individuals to use CGMs.

Immersive Virtual Reality or Immersive Virtual Alimentation and Nutrition (IVAN)

An area that is emerging in nutritional education and research is the use of virtual reality in conducting nutritional assessments. This technology allows users to interact with a virtual grocery store or kitchen setting to build their typical nutritional experience. A virtual setting can be beneficial if the individual cannot physically go to a grocery store or kitchen with the dietitian. The programs that are being developed can help individuals learn portion control, build meals, and apply knowledge in skill sessions or modules [12]. The use of this technology can be extended beyond research labs as it has the potential to address common barriers in traditional nutritional assessments and counseling. The use of programs like this in government support programs, clinics, schools, and individual homes will provide insight into individuals' behaviors and factors that may impact food choices.

The effectiveness of this newer technology is promising in the areas of practicing portion control, meal assembly, and food purchasing [12]. Education through actively practicing skills and building knowledge through conversations with dietitians or providers is essential. This program is currently limited and not yet publicly available; however, as technology continues to advance so will the exposure and use of this method.

Exploring the effectiveness of wearable devices and mobile applications in promoting healthy lifestyle behaviors and supporting nutritional management will evolve with technology. Current evidence to determine how these digital tools influence behavior change, improve health outcomes, and contribute to the nutritional assessment is important and can be another source of information to consider. Integration of technology into practical or clinical nutrition practice remains challenging. Barriers include clinician trust, safety and accuracy concerns, user engagement, and financial or resource limitations. However, behavioral integration shows more promising results. Wearables and mobile apps can deliver real-time feedback, reminders, and personalized guidance that help individuals translate biological signals into meaningful dietary and lifestyle changes. The current technology can capture behavior in naturalistic settings, enhancing adherence and long-term outcomes.

Advanced Biomarker Analysis

Another area of advancement is the broader use of biomarker analysis in the general population. Biomarkers are typically used in clinical settings to determine the scope of a certain disease or diagnosis of a disease state [13]. In nutritional assessment, the use of biomarker analysis can be beneficial for evaluating individual's intake of nutrients and non-nutritive foods as well as overall dietary patterns. Biomarkers can be broadly categorized into two key areas, molecular tools and biological characteristics, each offering valuable insights into the application and importance of these technologies.

Molecular Tools

The use of molecular biomarkers requires complex measures of various bodily fluids such as blood, urine, saliva, or tissues to be analyzed. This is considered an "omic" science, a high-throughput approach that uses advanced technologies to study entire biological system, providing insight into their structures, functions, pathways, and interactions [14]. Examples of how these tests can be used include genomics, proteomics, and metabolomics with most of the testing being done in laboratories and clinical settings. Genomics studies the entire DNA genome for structure, organization, and potential functions within the genes. Proteomics studies proteins in a cell or organism operation in various cellular processes. Metabolomics will utilize a biological sample to examine the end products of cellular processes or the current metabolic state. The various molecular tools will highlight the specific interconnection between health and disease at the cellular level. Currently, integrating the data from these three highlighted "omic" fields in general practice will be used for personalized medicine. Individuals can work with clinicians to examine disease risks, diagnose conditions earlier, and guide specific treatments for individuals [15]. Within nutritional assessment, personalized diets based on an individual's genetic and metabolic profile can optimize their health. Moreover, data could potentially prevent or manage chronic diseases like obesity, diabetes, and cardiovascular disease more effectively. This is a young area of research and application; however, further development of the field will foster standardization of testing and usage in the greater population.

Biological Characteristic Testing

Biomarker testing that will measure biological characteristics will utilize the "omic" data to provide further insights into the biological mechanisms and individual variations [16]. In essence, biological characteristics and testing are a broader field in which a sample will assess system-wide understanding of disease processes. The rationale for testing is hypothesized with a clear understanding of biological mechanisms. This broader approach could be a holistic approach that could combine traditional and molecular methods. For example, biological testing in nutrition assessment utilizes measurable indicators or biomarkers. These could include measuring blood glucose in diabetics, hemoglobin for iron status, and blood lipid panels to measure cholesterol. This type of testing can include functional, physiological, and genetic markers to identify specific needs and monitor the progression of diseases.

Technology has opened the opportunity for the general population to understand individual responses to food like gluten sensitivities and lactose intolerances. The rise of at-home testing that uses blood, urine, saliva, and stool can provide convenience and early detection of various biomarkers. More specifically, the use of antibody-based tests, DNA/RNA analysis, and biochemical assays can transform complex lab data into a user-friendly experience. The reliability and validity of at-home kits remain up for debate and should not be used to diagnosis any condition. User error is one of the largest factors that affects overall accuracy, with expiration dates and test type being other factors [17].

The use of advanced biomarker analysis will help personalize individual nutrition and diet by objectively measuring nutrient status, metabolic responses, and genetic variations. Gathering data and applying the information will help develop a personalized nutrition plan. For an individual, this might help identify vitamin or mineral deficiencies to then tailor supplements to address specific needs. Additionally, biomarkers can confirm whether changes to an individual's diet are having an impact on preventing disease or lowering disease risk. Combining the metabolic tools with the biological characteristics will strengthen the overall impact and drive strategies for optimal health.

Chapter Summary

This chapter explores how technology-driven tools are transforming nutritional assessment and enabling highly individualized approaches to diet and health. Modern assessment methods now extend far beyond traditional food records and anthropometrics, incorporating mobile apps, wearable devices, physiological sensors, and continuous glucose monitors (CGMs) to capture real-time data on eating patterns, activity levels, metabolic responses, and overall lifestyle behaviors. Emerging technologies such as Immersive Virtual Reality and Immersive Virtual Alimentation and Nutrition (IVAN) offer new ways to evaluate food choices, environmental influences, and behavioral responses in controlled yet realistic settings.

Advanced biomarker testing includes molecular tools, and biological characteristic analyses will add another layer of precision by identifying genetic, metabolic, and biochemical factors that influence nutrient needs and health outcomes. Together, these technologies provide a more complete picture of an individual's physiology, habits, and responses to dietary intake.

By integrating these data sources, nutrition professionals can tailor dietary recommendations with far greater accuracy. Personalized insights help identify optimal macronutrient distributions, detect nutrient deficiencies or excesses, monitor glycemic patterns, and adjust interventions based on objective and subjective feedback. Ultimately, technology-enhanced assessment supports a shift from generalized dietary guidelines to truly individualized nutrition strategies that improve health, performance, and long-term behavior change.

Chapter Review Questions

1. How do mobile apps and wearable devices enhance the accuracy and consistency of dietary and lifestyle tracking compared to traditional methods?
2. In what ways can continuous glucose monitors (CGMs) provide insights that support individualized nutrition planning?
3. Describe how immersive technologies such as IVAN can be used to assess eating behaviors in controlled yet realistic environments.
4. What types of information can advance biomarkers, such as molecular tools and biological characteristic testing, provide that traditional assessments cannot?
5. Discuss the potential challenges or limitations of relying on technology-driven assessments in nutrition practice.
6. Reflect on a scenario where technology might misrepresent or oversimplify an individual's nutritional needs. How should a practitioner respond?

References

1. Jospe MR, Fairbairn KA, Green P, Perry TL. Diet app use by sports dietitians: a survey in five countries. JMIR MHealth UHealth. 2015;3(1):e7. Available from: https://mhealth.jmir.org/2015/1/e7/
2. Morello O, McPhee L, Kucab M, Bellissimo N, Totosy de Zepetnek JO. Reliability and validity of nutrient assessment applications for Canadian endurance athletes: MyFitnessPal and Cronometer. J Hum Nutr Diet. 2025;38(5):e70148. https://doi.org/10.1111/jhn.70148.
3. Li RT, Kling SR, Salata MJ, Cupp SA, Sheehan J, Voos JE. Wearable performance devices in sports medicine. Sports Health. 2016;8(1):74–8. https://doi.org/10.1177/1941738115616917.
4. Jagim AR, Koch-Gallup N, Camic CL, Kroening L, Nolte C, Schroeder C, et al. The accuracy of fitness watches for the measurement of heart rate and energy expenditure during moderate intensity exercise. J Sports Med Phys Fitness. 2021;61(2):205–11. https://doi.org/10.23736/S0022-4707.20.11151-4.
5. Mattfeld R, Jesch E, Hoover A. Evaluating pedometer algorithms on semi-regular and unstructured gaits. Sensors (Basel). 2021;21(13):4260. https://doi.org/10.3390/s21134260.

6. Levine BD. VO2max: what do we know, and what do we still need to know?: maximal oxygen uptake. J Physiol. 2008;586(1):25–34. https://doi.org/10.1113/jphysiol.2007.147629.
7. Pasadyn SR, Soudan M, Gillinov M, Houghtaling P, Phelan D, Gillinov N, et al. Accuracy of commercially available heart rate monitors in athletes: a prospective study. Cardiovasc Diagn Ther. 2019;9(4):379–85. https://doi.org/10.21037/cdt.2019.06.05.
8. Fiore M, Bianconi A, Sicari G, Conni A, Lenzi J, Tomaiuolo G, et al. The use of smart rings in health monitoring—a meta-analysis. Appl Sci (Basel). 2024;14(23):10778. https://doi.org/10.3390/app142310778.
9. Kwon SY, Moon JS. Advances in continuous glucose monitoring: clinical applications. Endocrinol Metab (Seoul). 2025;40(2):161–73. https://doi.org/10.3803/EnM.2025.2370.
10. Mason LJ, Hartwig T, Greene D. Validating the use of continuous glucose monitors with nondiabetic recreational runners. Int J Sports Physiol Perform. 2024;19(11):1307–13. https://doi.org/10.1123/ijspp.2024-0102.
11. Klonoff DC, Nguyen KT, Xu NY, Gutierrez A, Espinoza JC, Vidmar AP. Use of continuous glucose monitors by people without diabetes: an idea whose time has come? J Diabetes Sci Technol. 2023;17(6):1686–97. https://doi.org/10.1177/19322968221110830.
12. Edwards CG, Sajjadi P, Fatemi A, Krieger EN, Klippel A, Masterson TD. The immersive virtual alimentation and nutrition application: an interactive digital dietitian. J Nutr Educ Behav. 2022;54(5):481–4. https://doi.org/10.1016/j.jneb.2022.02.014.
13. Picó C, Serra F, Rodríguez AM, Keijer J, Palou A. Biomarkers of nutrition and health: new tools for new approaches. Nutrients. 2019;11(5):1092. https://doi.org/10.3390/nu11051092.
14. Micheel CM, Nass SJ, Omenn GS. Board on Health Care Services, Board on health sciences policy, Omics-based clinical discovery: science, technology, and applications. Washington DC: National Academies Press; 2012.
15. Molla G, Bitew M. Revolutionizing personalized medicine: synergy with multi-omics data generation, main hurdles, and future perspectives. Biomedicines. 2024;12(12):2750. https://doi.org/10.3390/biomedicines12122750.
16. Graig LA, Phillips JK, Moses HL, et al. Committee on policy issues, board on health care services, introduction. Washington, DC: National Academies Press; 2016.
17. Salamon M. At-home tests: help or hindrance? [internet]. Harvard Health. 2023. Available from: https://www.health.harvard.edu/staying-healthy/at-home-tests-help-or-hindrance

Case Studies 10

Abstract

This chapter presents six case studies that illustrate diverse dietary journeys, designed to reinforce key concepts of nutritional assessment and the application of assessment tools. Rather than prescribing a single process, the case studies emphasize the importance of piecing together varied information to determine the most appropriate path for each individual. The case studies underscore the complexity of nutritional assessment, highlighting that no single standardized process exists; rather, practitioners must synthesize multiple sources of information to determine individualized pathways. The consistent framework across cases fosters a "learn by doing" approach, reinforcing theoretical concepts while encouraging analytical reasoning. Conducted individually or collaboratively, these exercises provide a learning environment for practicing assessment techniques, cultivating critical thinking, and appreciating diverse perspectives in nutritional evaluation.

Keywords

Estimated energy equations · Assessment · Food journal · Calories · Total calories

S. Kitts, *Nutritional Assessment*,
https://doi.org/10.1007/978-3-032-22506-1_10

Learning Objectives:
By the end of this chapter students should be able to:

- Analyze the nutritional status of the individual in each case by evaluating reported information such as basic demographics, patient specific data, food records or reported nutrient intakes, and use of estimated energy equations.
- Formulate a patient-focused assessment that connects results to current dietary guidelines.
- Evaluate potential barriers for individuals to make changes and suggestions for improving diet and physical activity.
- Differentiate between where education can be provided and the responsibilities of the health care team in the assessment.

This chapter will introduce six case studies that will highlight different individual's dietary journeys. The purpose of these case studies is to reinforce the concepts that have been discussed and the process of utilizing the assessment tools discussed. There is not one single process to follow, rather it is recognizing the pieces of the puzzle to determine the best path forward for an individual.

Each case study will follow the same layout to streamline the overarching concepts of nutritional assessment and support a 'learn-by-doing' approach that enhances critical thinking. Using the client background information, the data block containing key variables for calculations, and the dietary information provided or recorded, each case will represent real-world scenarios. There are times where an assessment might have imperfect or incomplete information, which is a crucial skill to navigate in case studies and real-world assessments. Essentially, these case studies offer a low-stake environment to practice decision-making and critical thinking when assessing an individual's health and dietary patterns. When these are done in groups, students will have a chance to discuss different perspectives and collaborate on how to approach nutritional assessment.

Considerations for all case studies should include:

- Background information that might give you information about the individual
- Using key variables to determine the best estimated energy equation to use
- Practicing interpretation of equation results and how they can be utilized
- Remembering the dietary guidelines and practices that all populations should consider
- Considering the areas that can be used to educate individuals on their dietary requirements and choices

Case studies require foundational knowledge to map the process of nutritional assessment. Each step can help you guide decisions or different pathways you might have to consider for an individual. Visualizing the process can help you see the alternative paths based on "yes" or "no" answers to specific diet or health questions. As you practice the decision-making process, it will help reduce uncertainty and increase logical steps to solving the individual's assessment puzzle. A visual map has been created to describe the possible sequence of steps (Diagram 10.1).

The flowchart gives a structural representation of the steps that need to happen to find an appropriate equation. However, understanding the positives and negatives of the individual equations can help streamline the assessment process. The following chart summarizes the equations discussed in Chap. 5 (Table 10.1).

This table is a good resource for the case studies as not all equations would be appropriate based on the individual-, background-, and patient-specific demographics. Again, there is no one specific equation that will work for everyone and your personal preferences might also influence your choice.

The following case studies were developed and cultivated from years of helping individuals with their nutritional journeys. Equations were picked for "best fit," and reasoning is provided based on information from peer-reviewed research. The purpose of these case studies is to help start conversations about approach-

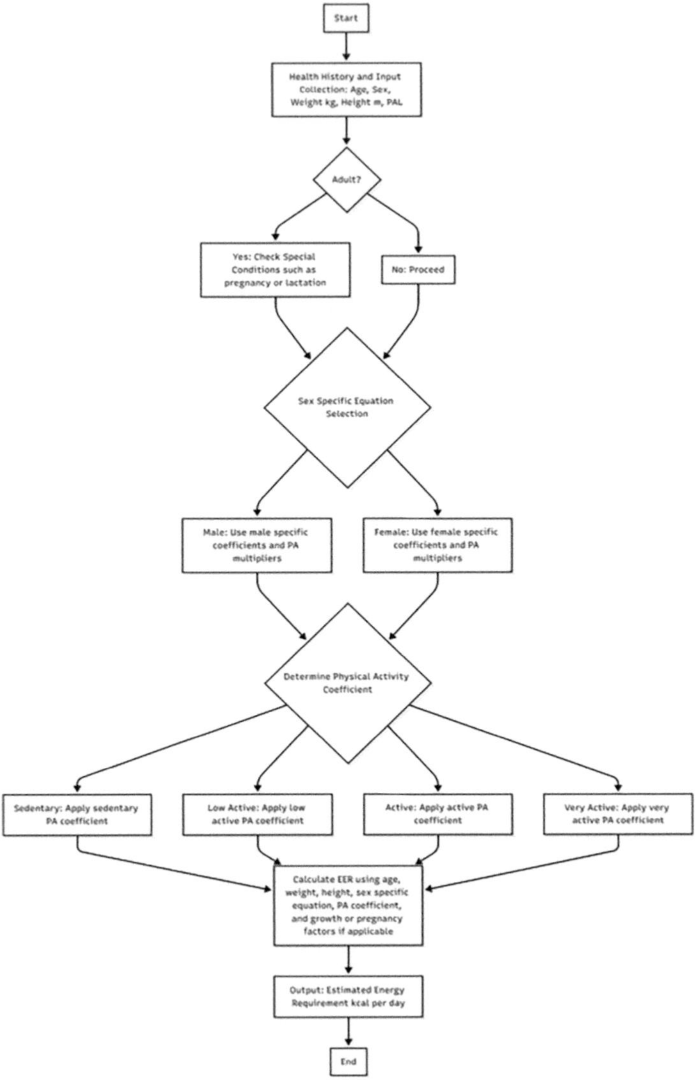

Diagram 10.1 A flowchart to visualize the steps to find an estimated energy equation

Table 10.1 Summary of the estimated energy equations used in specific populations

Equation	Population specificity	Population exclusions
Harris Benedict	Healthy normal weight adults	Overweight and obese
Mifflin St. Jeor	General population Gender-specific equation for adults	Less suitable for athletes, children, adolescents, or individuals with multiple comorbidities
Henry Oxford	Diverse population	Not appropriate for overweight or older population
Owen	Healthy normal weight adults	Overweight/obese, athlete/highly active, older population, children, adolescents, or individuals with multiple comorbidities
Schofield	Healthy population with normal weight (Western Europe and North American decent)	Not specific enough for obese individuals, those with underlying conditions, or global ethnic groups.
Katch-McArdle	Athletes and individuals with high physical activity	Obese individuals, older population, and medical conditions
Cunningham	Athletes (recreational or trained)	Sedentary lifestyle and individuals in a chronic disease state.

ing weight changes, the best way to assess calorie needs, and education about nutrient needs.

Case Study: Carbohydrate Overload

Background The individual has decided that he needed to make some changes to his diet and physical activity after being sedentary after an injury. In the past six months, he has joined a fitness facility and lost 15 lbs through aerobic activities such as running and elliptical training. He also lifts weights two times a week. He doesn't really have a plan for his diet; however, he has heard that he needs to be in a "calorie deficit" to lose weight. This individual would like to lose more weight but has recently hit a plateau.

Data Block:

Male – 36 y/o
- 6′2″ - Activity level – Moderate 1.65
- 195lbs - %BF – 28%
- Current reported calorie daily intake 2,475 calories

Food Journal:

Breakfast	Morning snack	Lunch	Mid-day snack	Dinner
2 servings of wheaties 2.5 cups of 1% milk 16 oz of orange juice	1 large egg bagel 2 Tbsp of peanut butter 2 12-oz cans of diet Pepsi	1 wheat sub-roll 4 oz of grilled chicken 2 Tbsp ranch dressing Mixed vegetables 2 12-oz cans of diet Pepsi 2 servings of Doritos (Nacho flavor)	2 12-oz cans of diet Pepsi	2 12-oz cans of diet Pepsi 1 16-oz strip steak 1.5 baked potatoes 2 strips of bacon 2 tbsp of sour cream 2 servings of macaroni and cheese

Assessment Strategies:

- Determine which equations you will use to assess the overall health and caloric need.
- Using the food journal as reference, what dietary patterns do you see or suggestions you would make for the individual to consider?
  – Highlight general nutrition recommendations to improve dietary outcomes.

Case Study: Carbohydrate Overload

Assessment Strategies

- *Calculate BMI*
  Height – 6′2″ → 74 inches × 0.0254 = 1.8796 m / 187.96 cm / 3.53 m^2

Weight – 195 lbs /2.2 = 88.64 kg
BMI = *kg*/*m*2
BMI = 88.64 kg / 3.53 m^2 = 25.11 kg/m^2 (Overweight classification)

- *Calculate BMR and TDEE (Mifflin St. Jeor)*
  (Males) RMR = (10 × weight in kg) + (6.25 × height in cm) – (5 × age in years) + 5
  RMR = (10 × 88.64 kg) + (6.25 × 187.96 cm) – (5 × 36) + 5
  RMR = (886.4) + (1,174.75) – (180) + 5
  RMR = 1,886.15 calories
  TDEE = RMR × PAL (activity level)
  TDEE = 1,886.15 × 1.65 = 3,112.15 calories
- *Additional Calculation of RMR and TEE to include FFM (Cunningham 1991)*
  FM = Total Body Weight (kg) × (Body Fat Percentage / 100)
  FM = 88.64 × (28%/100)
  FM = 88.64 × 0.28 = 24.82 kg
  LBM = Total Body Weight (kg) – Fat Mass (in kg)
  LBM = 88.64 – 24.82 = 63.82 kg
  RMR = 370 + 21.6 × FFM
  RMR = 370 + 21.6 × 63.82 kg = 1,748.51 calories
  TEE = 1,748.51 × PAL (activity level)
  TEE = 1,748.51 × 1.65 = 2,885.04 calories

Case Study: Carbohydrate Overload

Assessment Considerations:

- Equation findings
  - *BMI = 25.11 kg/m^2 (Overweight classification)*: By classification standards, the individual is currently overweight by the smallest margin. However, consideration should be given to the individual as he has lost 15 pounds, and his physical activity includes cardiovascular and strength training. It stands to reason that he has increased his overall muscle mass, and this could be a misclassification due to the equation not accounting for muscle mass, bone density,

or fat distribution or changes. This is an educational point to convey to the individual.

 - *BMR and TDEE (Mifflin St. Jeor)—RMR 1,886.15 calories, TDEE 3,112.15 calories*: The use of the Mifflin St. Jeor is appropriate as it is widely used to determine RMR in the general population, has age as a variable, and is a gender-specific equation. Additionally, this equation performs well with normal to obese weight individuals throughout the populations.
 - *RMR and TEE (Cunningham 1991)—RMR 1,748.51 calories, TEE 2,885.04 calories*: Using the Cunningham equation here is also appropriate as the individual has a reported %BF that could be applied. This is a bonus to have a reported %BF, as this is not always reported or feasible to obtain. As previously discussed, using FFM can be an independent predictor of RMR; therefore, using this equation could help assess and align goals of this individual.

 When comparing the results of these two formulas, the differences are minimal; RMR varies by 137.64 calories and TDEE/TEE varies by 227.11 calories. The energy equations are not a precise measure of an individual's metabolism, rather a predictive estimate. Using multiple estimates is not always needed; however, it can be beneficial to provide a starting point for planning diets, adjusting, and meeting the individual's goals.

- Equation Assessment
 - The equations for this individual show that he is making some dietary changes that would initiate weight loss. If you add back the 15-pound weight loss to his new weight, he weighed 210 pounds when he started, his BMI then was 27.04 kg/m^2. Decreasing his BMI by two points will help decrease health risks and increase quality of life. Both energy equations account for important variables; Mifflin St. Jeor uses the variables of age, gender, and activity level, and Cunningham uses the FFM component to better predict caloric need. Therefore, using the ranges of total calories can be beneficial for this individual if they want to continue

to lose weight by decreasing calories under the current predictions. If the individual wanted to maintain weight, he would use the predicted values.

Case Study: Carbohydrate Overload

Nutritional Assessment Plan

- *Medical History*—collect information on weight history and family history.
- *Physical Activity*—inquire about hours training per week and intensity levels.
- *Physical exam*—clinician will perform a physical exam (measuring blood pressure, heart rate).
- *Diet assessment*—current reported food journal needs refocusing on variety of dense carbohydrates and lean proteins. Education about good sources of nutrients, increased fiber for their age, and decreasing the about of processed foods would help. Changes like this might complement additional weight loss.

Goal Setting or Habit Identification

- After reviewing a client's nutritional analysis, what steps would you take to identify their current eating habits and create personalized goals that support sustainable dietary change?

Case Study: Possible Eating Disorder Assessment

Background Lydia is an 18-year-old freshman college gymnast at an out-of-state university. She weighs 88 lbs and her athletic physical revealed he body fat % to be 11%. She trains for 3 hours and has a training calorie of 511cal. Lydia wants to be an athlete all 4 years of college, so when a few friends told her to see a dietitian to make sure she stayed healthy in season since she seemed a little too thin, she went ahead and saw the university's dietitian. The Registered Dietitian requested a food journal and asked Lydia what her relationship with food was like, where Lydia revealed she was a pescetarian and since moving away from home struggled to find meals that followed her dietary needs.

Data Block:

Female gymnast - 18y/o

- 4'9"
- 88lbs
- %BF – 11%
- Training Calories – 511cal
- In season – 3 hour practices (PAL 1.725)

Food Journal

Please analyze the athlete's diet for overall calories and variety in nutrients.

Breakfast	16 oz cranberry juice 1 cup cornflakes or rice crispies 6 oz skim milk	381 calories
Mid-morning	8oz green tea 1 medium-sized apple	74 calories
Lunch	16 oz water 1 hardboiled egg 1 ½ cups spinach 5 grape tomatoes ½ cup carrot (shredded) 1 tbsp fat-free Italian dressing	104 calories
Dinner	1 ½ cup wheat pasta 1 tbsp of butter ½ cup peas ¼ cup tuna fish ½ cup rice pudding 8 oz low-fat chocolate milk	730 calories

Current diet: 1,289 total calories

Assessment Strategies:

- Determine which equations you will use to assess the overall health and caloric need.
- Using the food journal as reference, what dietary patterns do you see or suggestions you would make for the athlete to consider?

Case Study: Possible Eating Disorder Assessment

Assessment Strategies:

- *Calculate BMI*

  Height – 4′9″ → 57 inches × 0.0254 = 1.4478 m / 144.78 cm / 2.096 m^2

  Weight – 88lbs / 2.2 = 40kg

  BMI = *kg/m2*

  BMI = 40kg/2.096 m^2 = 19.08 kg/m^2 (Healthy classification)
- *Calculate BMR and TDEE (Katch-McArdle)*
  - Calculate Fat Mass: Fat Mass (in kg) = Total Body Weight (kg) × (Body Fat Percentage / 100)
  - Calculate Lean Body Mass: Lean Body Mass (in kg) = Total Body Weight (kg) – Fat Mass (in kg).
  - BMR= 370 + (21.6 × lean body mass (kg))
  - Utilize PAL to determine TDEE

  FM = 40kg × (11% × 100)

  FM = 40kg × 0.11 = 4.4kg

  LBM = 40kg – 4.4kg = 35.6kg

  BMR= 370 + (21.6 × lean body mass (kg))

  BMR = 370 + (21.6 × 35.6kg)

  BMR = 370 + (768.96)

  BMR = 1138.96 calories

  TDEE = BMR × PAL (activity level)

  TDEE = 1138.9 × 1.725 = 1964.71 calories

Case Study: Possible Eating Disorder Assessment

- *Calculate Energy Availability*
  - Athletes' kg – %BF = LBM
  - Energy intake – training calories = Residual energy
  - Residual energy / LBM = Energy availability
  - Compare to critical cutoff—is it appropriate for athlete

  40kg – 11% (4.4) = 35.6 kg LBM

  1,289 – 511 = 778 Residual Energy

  778/35.6 = 21.85 Energy Availability

  21.85 Below Critical Cutoff

Assessment Considerations:

- Equation findings
  - *BMI = 40kg/2.096 m² = 19.08 kg/ m² (Healthy classification)*: By classification standards, the athlete has a healthy BMI classification; however, it is on the lower end of the healthy range. In cases like this, it is advisable to monitor the athlete for potential health concerns and changes in hormonal disruption. Therefore, an energy-availability assessment and a dietary assessment should be conducted together to ensure that sufficient calories are available to support both performance and overall health.
  - *BMR and TDEE (Katch-McArdle)—BMR 1,138.96 calories, TDEE 1,964.71 calories*: Use of the Katch-McArdle equation is appropriate for this athlete because of a high muscle mass, consideration of LBM, and the ability to provide a more accurate BMR to align daily caloric needs for training, recovery, and performance.

    Specifically, to this athlete, the equation establishes the baseline calories needed (1,138.96) and total calories to support activity (1,964.71). The reported food journal captures on day of 1,289 total calories which is slightly above the determined BMR and well below the determined 1,964.71. This could be a concern for the athlete if they are not taking enough calories to support the physical activity demand, therefore creating an energy deficit. This could be a one-day anomaly or a case of underreporting; in either case, it should be addressed as an educational topic when discussing the athlete's overall diet.
  - *Energy Availability—21.85 kcal/kg FFM/Day Below Critical Cutoff*: The result here is below the critical cutoff of 45 kcal/kg FFM/day, which is the general accepted optimal range for energy availability. This finding should be used as one indicator, not the sole indicator that the athlete may be in a calorie deficit. A further assessment of the athlete's overall health, diet, and activity levels will need to be done, not the result of the equation.

- Equation Assessment
  - The three results of the equations could indicate that the athlete is in an energy deficit and should consider increasing calories accounting for activity calories. Using these equations together, rather than stand-alone results, is more meaningful and helps to support the nutritional assessment.

Nutritional Assessment Plan

- *Medical History*—collect information on weight history, signs and symptoms (fatigue, frequent colds/illness, menstrual history), and family history.
- *Physical Activity*—inquire about training load (in or out of season), hours training per week, and if training load has increased or decreased.
- *Physical exam*—clinician will perform a physical exam (measuring blood pressure, heart rate). Communication and referral to health care team is advised.
- *Diet assessment*—Current reported food journals lack calories, diversity of carbohydrate and protein sources, and calories needed for recovery. Education to increase variety and ensure adequate intake can help maintain performance goals, prevent injuries, and support immune function.

Goal Setting or Habit Identification

- After reviewing a client's nutritional analysis, what steps would you take to identify their current eating habits and create personalized goals that support sustainable dietary change?

Case Study: Weight Loss Confusion

Background: Mrs. D is a 40-year-old mother of three. She has arthritis in both knees. She weighs 180 pounds, has a medium frame, and is 5 ft 3 in. tall. Her physician has told her to lose weight to help reduce her knee pain. According to Mrs. D, she never thought that she was overweight until she was 24 years old. At this time, her weight started increasing. When she weighed 140 pounds, she started to diet. One time she lost a total of 25 pounds, which she promptly regained plus an additional 5 pounds. She described four additional weight loss cycles. Mrs. D claims that she cannot exercise because "it is too painful on my knees." She has tried every conceivable type of diet, including a comprehensive medically supervised weight-control program. Mrs. D states that for the past year, no matter how little she eats, she cannot lose weight even on a 1,200-kilocalorie diet.

Data Block:

Female – 40 y/o - 5'3" - Activity level – Low (1.2) - 180lbs

Food Journal

Analyze Mrs. D's diet using a two-day food journal. Please note homemade is designated by (H) and packaged/processed will be (P) as this is something her dietitian wanted her to focus on.

DAY 1		Day 2	
Breakfast (239 calories, 26 g protein)	1 cup raspberries 1 cup nonfat plain Greek yogurt 1 Tbsp. sliced almonds	Breakfast (230 calories, 11 g protein)	1 Serving egg salad avocado toast (H)
A.M. Snack (64 calories, 1 g protein)	1 cup raspberries	A.M. Snack (64 calories, 1 g protein)	1 Cup raspberries
Lunch (519 calories, 34 g protein)	1 Serving chicken quinoa bowl with olives and cucumber (H)	Lunch (519 calories, 34 g protein)	1 Serving chicken quinoa bowl with olives and cucumber (H)
P.M. Snack (42 calories, 1 g protein)	1 kiwi	P.M. Snack (62 calories, 1 g protein)	1 Medium orange
Dinner (348 calories, 24 g protein)	1 lean cuisine Asian beef noodle bowl (P)	Dinner (351 calories, 33 g protein)	1 Healthy choice spicy jerk shrimp (P)

DAY 1		Day 2	
Daily Totals: 1,212 calories, 87 g protein, 112 g carbohydrates, 27 g fiber, 47 g fat, 1,265 mg sodium		Daily Totals: 1,225 calories, 81 g protein, 116 g carbohydrates, 26 g fiber, 50 g fat, 1,502 mg sodium	

Assessment Strategies:

- Determine which equations you will use to assess overall health and caloric need.
- Using the food journal as reference, what dietary patterns do you see or suggestions you would make for the individual to consider?

Case Study: Weight Loss Confusion

Assessment Strategies:

- *Calculate BMI*
  Height – 5′3″ ➔ 63 inches × 0.0254 = 1.6002 m / 160.02 cm / 2.56 m^2
  Weight – 180lbs / 2.2 = 81.82kg
  BMI = *kg/m2*
  BMI = 81.82kg/2.56 m^2 = 31.96 kg/m^2 (Obese classification)
- *Calculate BMR and TDEE (Mifflin St. Jeor)*
  (Females) RMR = (10 × weight in kg) + (6.25 × height in cm) – (5 × age in years) – 161
  RMR = (10 × 81.82) + (6.25 × 160.02) – (5 × 40) – 161
  RMR = (818.2) + (1,000.125) – (200) – 161
  RMR = 1,457.32 calories
  TDEE = RMR × PAL (activity level)
  TDEE = 1,457.32 × 1.2 = 1,748.78 calories

Assessment Considerations:

- Equation findings
  - *BMI = 31.96 kg/m^2 (Obese classification)*: By classification standards, the individual is obese and can be further categorized as class 1 obesity. Individuals with BMI of 30 or above have a higher risk of developing health problems such as

type 2 diabetes, high blood pressure, and heart disease. Although she has had issues with weight gain on a reduced calorie diet, she also explained that there were several weight cycles where she would lose and then gain weight back. Continuing guidance from her health care team will be recommended.
  - *BMR and TDEE (Mifflin St. Jeor) = RMR 1,457.32 calories, TDEE 1,748.78 calories*: The use of the Mifflin St. Jeor is appropriate as it is widely used to determine RMR in the general population as this equation performs well with normal to obese weight individuals throughout the populations. In this instance, due to her lack of physical activity or sedentary lifestyle, the RMR will account for the larger part of the total calories burned daily.

Case Study: Weight Loss Confusion

- Equation Assessment
  - The results from the two equations point to a combination of factors that include a sedentary lifestyle, possible metabolic adaptations through a history of dieting, and potential hormonal and metabolic disorders. Continued work and monitoring with her health care team is advised.

Nutritional Assessment Plan

- *Medical History*—collect information on weight history, signs and symptoms of any disease states, and family history.
- *Physical Activity*—inquire about low-impact exercises like swimming, water aerobics, cycling, and yoga/tai chi to limit impact on joints. Low intensity exercises can help to reduce stress and help increase physical activity.
- *Physical exam*—clinician will perform a physical exam (measuring blood pressure, heart rate). In addition, ordering laboratory tests like lipid panels, glucose, and thyroid function tests could be beneficial.

- *Diet assessment*—Current reported food journal already being assessed and monitored by dietician. Support could be given by discussing how to build the importance of increasing fruits, vegetables, and fiber. Additionally, limiting processed or easily prepared foods can help with overall dietary ownership of nutrients.

Goal Setting or Habit Identification

- After reviewing a client's nutritional analysis, what steps would you take to identify their current eating habits and create personalized goals that support sustainable dietary change?

Case Study: Protein Diet Confusion

Background: Denise is a 24-year-old female. She has been following a high-protein weight loss regimen for two months after watching an infomercial on this type of weight-loss diet. In this diet, the claim is that protein complementation is achieved for overall weight loss. To properly track progression, an app is advised to monitor overall protein intake and weight loss.

Denise loves to eat fast food and sweets, a diet that has caused her to gain excess body weight and fat. When asked about it, she says her usual way of eating needs to change, so she is on a diet. The change in her food selection has caused her to eliminate the intake of all fruits, grain products, starchy vegetables, legumes, and refined baked goods, as well as nearly eliminate the intake of dairy products such as milk, yogurt, and ice cream. As a result, she consumes a lot of meat, cheese, nuts, olives, and diet Jell-O. Because she doesn't like the taste of water, she is drinking mostly caffeinated diet soda.

Most of her calories are from fat (55 percent of total calories are from fat, with a high intake of saturated fatty acids and cholesterol), a high level from protein (35 percent of total calories), and a low intake level of carbohydrates (10 percent of calories). Her diet was analyzed and found to be extremely deficient in calories, dietary fiber, and many water-soluble vitamins and some major and trace minerals.

Data Block:

Female – 24 y/o
- 5'5"   - Activity level – Low (1.2)
- 165lbs

Diet Plan: *Example of the high-protein weight-loss regimen patient found online*

"We designed this meal plan to provide you with plenty of variety. However, feel free to swap out recipes based on your food preferences for meals that suit your lifestyle and cooking preferences. For example, if you find a breakfast you love—such as our keto egg and bacon casserole—go ahead and eat it every morning if you like.

Each day provides more than 100 grams of protein and less than 26 grams of net carbs."

Day 1	Day 2
Calories—1,634	Calories – 1,597
Fat—99.85 grams	Fat – 97.59 grams
Protein—142.97 grams	Protein—139.74 grams
Carbohydrate—40.85 grams	Carbohydrates—39.93 grams
Sodium—1,275 mg	Sodium—930 mg
Fiber—16 grams	Fiber—20 grams

Case Study: Protein Diet Confusion

Assessment Strategies:

- Determine which equations you will use to assess the overall health and caloric need.
- Using dietary analysis from an app and reported information as reference, what dietary patterns do you see or suggestions you would make for the individual to consider.
  - Comparison to dietary guidelines should be utilized and part of educational recommendations.

Assessment Strategies:

- *Calculate BMI*
  Height – 5′5″ → 65 inches × 0.0254 = 1.651 m / 165.10 cm / 2.725 m^2
  Weight – 165lbs / 2.2 = 75 kg
  BMI = *kg/m2*
  BMI = 75kg / 2.725 m^2 = 27.52 kg/m^2 (Overweight classification)
- *Calculate BMR and TDEE (Mifflin St. Jeor)*
  (Females) RMR = (10 × weight in kg) + (6.25 × height in cm) – (5 × age in years) – 161
  RMR = (10 × 75 kg) + (6.25 × 165.10 cm) – (5 × 24) – 161
  RMR = (750) + (1,031.875) – 120 – 161
  RMR = 1,500.875 calories
  TDEE = RMR × PAL (Activity level)
  TDEE = 1,500.875 × 1.2 = 1801.05 calories

Assessment Considerations:

- Equation findings
  - *BMI = 27.52 kg/m^2 (Overweight classification)*: By classification standards, the individual is overweight and by reevaluating her diet could help with lowering her BMI. Implementing a plan that includes physical activity through walking or other movements could help weight loss while preserving lean body mass and muscles.
  - *BMR and TDEE (Mifflin St. Jeor) = RMR 1,500.87 calories, TDEE 1801.05 calories*: The use of the Mifflin St. Jeor is appropriate as it is used for general populations to gauge everyday nutrition. Age, height, and weight are provided, making the calculation feasible to assess the individual's caloric need.

Case Study: Protein Diet Confusion

For this individual, they are reporting a daily total calorie intake close to RMR. The individual is young and reports no physical activity currently. When the total calorie intake is close to RMR during a weight loss cycle, the body may conserve energy leading to slower weight loss, fatigue, potential muscle loss, and weight loss plateaus.

- Equation Assessment
  - The results from the two equations show that there is some room for improvement in the individual's diet and activity level that would support further weight loss. The current weight-loss plan is unsustainable due to the severe caloric restriction and unbalanced nutrient intake.

Nutritional Assessment Plan

- *Medical History*—collect information on weight history, signs and symptoms of any disease states, and family history.
- *Physical Activity*—inquire about whether adding low-impact exercises can be impactful on weight loss as extra calories will be utilized. Combining calorie reduction with activities such as light strength training and adequate protein sources can signal the body to maintain muscle.
- *Physical exam*—clinician will perform a physical exam (measuring blood pressure, heart rate). In addition, ordering laboratory tests like lipid panels, glucose, and thyroid function tests could be beneficial. Additionally, hormonal shifts in cortisol, ghrelin, leptin, and others can vary as the body tries to conserve energy due to caloric deficits.
- *Diet assessment*—Current reported food journal has areas of improvement as indicated by current dietary guidelines. Education discussing how to increase fruits, vegetables, and fiber is important to support protein usage in weight loss.

Goal Setting or Habit Identification

- After reviewing a client's nutritional analysis, what steps would you take to identify their current eating habits and create personalized goals that support sustainable dietary change?

Case Study: Making Changes

Background: John has recently decided that he needs to lose weight because he was diagnosed as being prediabetic. This reality check has John motivated him to lose weight and get healthier. He has started to increase his physical activity by walking five days a week with his wife and strength training three times a week at a gym. John also bought a scale that provides him with his weight and body fat, he has not had a professional assessment to be more valid. You want to show John that he needs to eat more consciously and be aware of what he is eating. You decide to focus on one day that he consumed a total of 2518 calories. John only provides a screenshot of an app that he uses to track his daily macronutrients and does not provide a food journal or record. With this limited information you can use the macronutrient daily grams to examine his macronutrient distribution and compare it to current guidelines for the population. John believes that he is doing a fair job with his diet; however, there are changes that can be made to help him achieve his goals.

Data Block:

Male – 42 y/o

- 6'1" - Activity level – Moderate 1.8
- 235lbs - %BF – 30%
- Current reported calorie daily intake 2,518 cal

Reported food macronutrient grams from app:

Carbohydrates: 217g
Protein: 75 g
Fat: 150g

Assessment Strategies:

- Determine which equations you will use to assess the overall health and caloric need.
- Using dietary analysis from an app, what suggestions you would make for the individual to consider.
  - Comparison to dietary guidelines should be utilized and part of educational recommendations.
- Determine the macronutrient ratios to understand where the distribution of calories is coming from.

Case Study: Making Changes

Assessment Strategies:

- *Calculate BMI*
  Height – 6′1″ → 73 inches × 0.0254 = 1.854 m / 185.42 cm / 3.428 m^2
  Weight – 235lbs / 2.2 = 106.81 kg
  BMI = *kg/m2*
  BMI = 106.81 kg / 3.43 m^2 = 31.13 kg/m^2 (Obese classification)
- *Calculate BMR and TDEE (Mifflin St. Jeor)*
  (Males) RMR = (10 × weight in kg) + (6.25 × height in cm) – (5 × age in years) + 5
  RMR = (10 × 106.81 kg) + (6.25 × 185.42 cm) – (5 × 42) + 5
  RMR = (1068.1) + (1,158.875) – (210) + 5
  RMR = 2,021.97 calories
  TDEE = RMR × PAL (Activity level)
  TDEE = 2,021.97 × 1.8 = 3,639.55 calories
  Calculate Macronutrient Ratio Distribution
  Carbohydrates—217 grams × 4kcal = 868 calories / 2,518 total calories × 100 = **34.47%**
  Proteins—75 grams × 4kcal = 300 calories / 2,518 total calories × 100 = **11.91%**
  Fats—150 grams × 9kcal = 1,350 calories / 2,518 total calories × 100 = **53.61%**

Assessment Considerations:

- Equation findings
  - *BMI = 31.13 kg/m² (Obese classification)*: By classification standards, the individual is obese and can be further categorized under Class 1 Obesity. With his current diagnosis of prediabetic and his BMI classification, the individual might be at a higher risk of type 2 diabetes, high blood pressure, heart disease, and further progression of diabetic status.. Lifestyle and dietary changes are recommended.

Case Study: Making Changes

- *BMR and TDEE (Mifflin St. Jeor) = RMR 2,021.97 calories, TDEE 3,639.55 calories*: The use of this equation is appropriate; however, caution should be used as research has shown that accuracy declines slightly when assessing individuals with BMIs higher than 30. Since the individual is actively trying to lose weight, this equation is the most appropriate and should be monitored when weight loss happens.
- *Macronutrient Ratio Distribution—Carbohydrate 34% / Protein 11% / Fat 53%*: The macronutrient distribution range can be very helpful in determining areas of concern or potential for change within the diet. Manipulating the ratios can help with managing weight changes by highlighting the nutrients needed to provide energy and satiety or fullness while still creating a calorie deficit for weight loss.
- Equation Assessment
  - The results from the equations provide feedback to the health care team on where changes can be made to help with weight management for this individual. The Mifflin St. Jeor and macronutrient ratio distribution results could be an area to focus on as the individual is already creating a calorie deficit; however, potential redistribution of macronutrients could help with additional weight loss. Adjustment of macronutrients may create a more sustainable diet by increasing protein (for satiety), strategic emphasis on fiber

carbohydrates (for energy and overall health), and moderation of healthy fats (focusing on unsaturated).

Nutritional Assessment Plan

- *Medical History*—collect information on weight history, signs and symptoms of any disease states, and family history.
- *Physical Activity*—aim for consistent daily exercise that combines cardiovascular aerobic activities such as walking or cycling with strength training. The combination of these activities will help by increasing caloric output and maintaining muscle to increase metabolic output.
- *Physical exam*—clinician will perform a physical exam (measuring blood pressure, heart rate). In addition, ordering laboratory tests like lipid panels, glucose, and thyroid function tests could be beneficial. Additionally, due to prediabetic diagnosis, health care team should monitor blood sugar through regular A1C testing.
- *Diet assessment*—The results from the Mifflin St. Jeor and macronutrient ratio distribution offer the largest opportunity to educate the individual on dietary changes. As described, the individual is currently reporting 2,518 calories which is below the

Case Study: Making Changes

Estimated TDEE of 3,639.55 calories. This deficit in calories will promote weight loss and there is no need for the estimated high calories. The macronutrient ratio does not align with current guidelines for the general population, most evident in 53% of calories coming from fat versus the guideline of 30% or less.

For this individual, dietary adjustments might include limiting saturated fats, sugar, and refined carbs, and incorporate healthy fats and lean protein sources. Consideration for redistributing macronutrients to the 40/30/30 (carbs/protein/fats) split into a starting point could help balancing energy, satiety, and nutrition goals.

Goal Setting or Habit Identification

- After reviewing a client's nutritional analysis, what steps would you take to identify their current eating habits and create personalized goals that support sustainable dietary change?

Case Study: Preseason Athlete

Background: Collegiate male basketball is seeking to understand how to add weight before the season starts. His training schedule includes cardiovascular/cross-training workouts and strength training three times/week. Specifically, he would like to increase his lean body mass (11lbs) to challenge himself for a starting position. Recently started taking whey protein (22 g of protein, 2 g of carbohydrate per serving) as members of his team said it could help. He has no experience in kitchen, doesn't cook for himself, and usually grabs food on the go. He eats three meals a day and snacks are inconsistent. After a quick review of a food journal record from an app, it is determined that the current macronutrient ratios range from 50–55% CHO, 25–30% FAT, 17–20% PRO.

Data Block:

Male – 19 y/o	
- 6′7″	- Activity level – Active 1.54
- 196lbs	- %BF – 19%
	- Training calories = 775

Food Journal from app: (2,815 calories)

Breakfast	Grab & Go from Cafeteria Egg sandwich (1 scrambled egg, 1 slice of 2% cheddar cheese, 1 whole wheat English Muffin) 1 cup of 1% milk
Morning Snack	From Training Table 1 cup of grapes 6 oz. low-fat vanilla yogurt with ¼ cup of granola cereal

Lunch	Grab & Go from Cafeteria Chicken Caesar pita (1/2 grilled chicken breast, 2 romaine lettuce leaves, 2 slices of tomato, 4 slices cucumber, 2 tbsp Caesar salad dressing, 1 tbsp parmesan cheese) 1 medium orange ½ cup goldfish crackers 8 oz 1% milk
Afternoon snack	1 cup applesauce: Dorm room
Dinner	Main Cafeteria Stir-fry (5 oz. sirloin steak, 1 cup brown rice, ½ green pepper, 10 sugar snap peas, and 1 cup of broccoli) 16 oz water
Evening Snack	2 cups of tortilla chips and 1 cup thick and chunky salsa 8 oz 1% milk: Dorm room
During Practice	60 ounces of Powerade

Assessment Strategies:

- Determine which equations you will use to assess the overall health and caloric need.
- Using dietary analysis from an app, what suggestions you would make for the individual to consider.
- What special considerations should be accounted for with this individual?

Case Study: Preseason Athlete

Assessment Strategies:

- *Calculate BMI*

  Height: 6′7″ ➔ 79 inches × 0.0254 = 2.006 m / 200.66 cm / 4.026 m^2

  Weight: 196 lbs / 2.2 = 89.091 kg

  BMI = *kg/m2*

  BMI = 89.091 kg / 4.026 m^2 = 22.13 kg/m^2 (Normal or Health Classification)

- *Calculate BMR and TDEE (Katch-McArdle)*
  - Calculate Fat Mass: Fat Mass (in kg) = Total Body Weight (kg) × (Body Fat Percentage / 100)
  - Calculate Lean Body Mass: Lean Body Mass (in kg) = Total Body Weight (kg) – Fat Mass (in kg).
  - BMR= 370 + (21.6 × lean body mass (kg))
  - Utilize PAL to determine TDEE

  FM = 89.09kg × (19% × 100)
  FM = 89.09kg × 0.19 = 16.93kg
  LBM = 89.09kg – 16.93kg = 72.16kg
  BMR = 370 + (21.6 × LBM kg)
  BMR = 370 + (21.6 × 72.16kg)
  BMR = 370 + (1,558.65)
  BMR = 1,928.66 calories
  TDEE = BMR × PAL (Activity level)
  TDEE = 1,928.66 × 1.54 = 2,9070.13 calories

Case Study: Preseason Athlete

- *Calculate Energy Availability*
  - Athletes' kg – %BF = LBM
  - Energy intake – training calories = Residual energy
  - Residual energy / LBM = Energy availability
  - Compare to critical cutoff—is it appropriate for athlete

  89.09kg – 19% (16.93kg) = 72.16 kg
  2,815 – 775 = 2,040 Residual Energy
  2,040/72.16 = 28.27 Energy Availability
  28.27 Below Critical Cutoff

Assessment Considerations:

- Equation findings
  - *BMI = 22.13 kg/m² (Normal or Health Classification)*: By classification standards, the individual is a normal or healthy person. This can signify an ideal body type for active sports as the individual has lean muscle mass tissue and no excess fat tissue. However, this result should be used as a guideline

as it is more important to assess other metrics that can account for muscle mass.
  - *BMR and TDEE (Katch-McArdle) = BMR 1,928.66 calories, TDEE 2,9070.13 calories*: This equation is appropriate for athletic populations because it provides a tailored estimate of metabolic rate based on lean body mass. The additional variable of %BF will provide a more accurate estimate of calories as athletes generally have more muscle mass.
  - *Energy Availability = 28.27 Below Critical Cutoff*: The result here is below the critical cutoff of 45 kcal/kg FFM/day of the general accepted optimal range for energy availability. This finding should be used as another indicator, not a sole indicator, that the athlete might be in a calorie deficit. Examining the preseason training load will help optimize nutrition and the goal of increasing muscle mass for this individual.
- Equation Assessment
  - The results from the equations will help make some strategic changes to support the individual's activity as well as goal to increase muscle mass in the preseason. Although the individual is reporting a current intake of 2,815 calories which is close to the result of the estimated caloric intake (estimated 2,9070 calories), there is room to increase energy intake. Additionally, if calories are increased, it would be protective against low energy availability.

Case Study: Preseason Athlete

Nutritional Assessment Plan

- *Medical History*—collect information on weight history, signs and symptoms of any disease states, and family history.
- *Physical Activity*—assess current training load and account for preseason training increases. Caloric output may be higher as training during preseason sometimes entails multiple training times that could include cardiovascular and strength training on the same day.

- *Physical exam*—clinician will perform a physical exam (measuring blood pressure, heart rate). Referral to registered dietitians on campus is advised.
- *Diet assessment*—continue to track individual's food journal and implement strategic fueling. To achieve this, meals and snacks should be planned to ensure fuel for activity and basic body function. Choosing energy-dense, nutrient-rich foods should be the basis of diet and liquid nutrition to supplement additional calories. Also, education for the individual on how to navigate the cafeterias on campus and what to buy for the dorm room can maximize calories.

Goal Setting or Habit Identification

- After reviewing a client's nutritional analysis, what steps would you take to identify their current eating habits and create personalized goals that support sustainable dietary change?

Chapter Summary

This chapter provides a structured exploration of nutritional assessment through the application of six case studies. Each Case Study is designed to replicate real-world scenarios, thereby reinforcing theoretical concepts and fostering the development of practical skills. The overarching aim is to cultivate critical thinking and decision-making abilities in the evaluation of individual dietary patterns and health status. The pedagogical design of the chapter emphasizes experiential learning. By engaging in case-based analysis, students practice synthesizing diverse forms of information to construct meaningful assessments. Group work further enhances this process by encouraging dialogue, collaboration, and the consideration of multiple perspectives. Ultimately, the chapter underscores that nutritional assessment is not a prescriptive formula but a dynamic process of integrating diverse data points to determine the most appropriate course of action for everyone.

Chapter Review Questions

1. How can demographic information, patient-specific data, food records, and estimated energy equations be integrated to evaluate an individual's nutritional status?
2. In what ways can the results of a nutritional assessment be connected to current dietary guidelines to formulate a patient-focused plan?
3. What are common barriers individuals may face when attempting to change dietary or physical activity habits, and what strategies can be suggested to overcome these barriers?
4. How can the responsibilities of the health care team be distinguished from opportunities for patient education during the assessment process?
5. Explain how habit identification and goal setting can be integrated into the nutritional assessment process to help individuals translate assessment findings into meaningful, long-term behavior change.

Index

S. Kitts, *Nutritional Assessment*,
https://doi.org/10.1007/978-3-032-22506-1

MIX
Papier aus verantwortungsvollen Quellen
Paper from responsible sources
FSC® C105338

If you have any concerns about our products,
you can contact us on
ProductSafety@springernature.com

In case Publisher is established outside the EU,
the EU authorized representative is:
Springer Nature Customer Service Center GmbH
Europaplatz 3, 69115 Heidelberg, Germany

Printed by Libri Plureos GmbH
in Hamburg, Germany